The Comfort
of Home™
for Stroke

A Guide for Caregivers

The Comfort of Home caregiver book series is written for family and paraprofessional home caregivers who face the responsibilities of caring for aging friends, family, or clients. The disease-specific editions, often in collaboration with organizations supporting those conditions, address caregivers assisting people with those diseases.

Other Caregiver Resources from CareTrust Publications:

The Comfort of Home™: *A Complete Guide for Caregivers—Third Edition*
La comodidad del hogar™ *(Spanish Edition)*
The Comfort of Home™ *Multiple Sclerosis Edition*
The Comfort of Home™ *for Parkinson Disease: A Guide for Caregivers*
The Comfort of Home™ *for Chronic Lung Disease: A Guide for Caregivers*
The Comfort of Home™ *for Alzheimer's Disease: A Guide for Caregivers*
The Comfort of Home™ *Caregiving Journal*
The Comfort of Home™ *Caregivers—Let's Take Care of You!* Meditation CD

Newsletters:

The Comfort of Home™ *Caregiver Assistance News*
The Comfort of Home™ *Grand-Parenting News*
The Comfort of Home™ *Caregivers—Let's Take Care of You!*

Visit www.comfortofhome.com for forthcoming editions and other caregiver resources.

The Comfort of Home™ for Stroke

A Guide for Caregivers

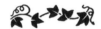

Maria M. Meyer

and

Paula Derr, RN, BSN, CEN, CCRN

with

Jon Caswell, *Stroke Connection Magazine*

CareTrust Publications LLC
"Caring for you...caring for others."
Portland, Oregon

The Comfort of Home™ for Stroke: A Guide for Caregivers

Copyright © 2007 Maria M. Meyer

Published by: CareTrust Publications LLC
P.O. Box 10283
Portland, Oregon 97296-0283
(800) 565-1533
Fax (503) 221-7019

Publisher's Cataloging-in-Publication
(Provided by Quality Books, Inc.)

Meyer, Maria M., 1948-
    The comfort of home for Stroke : a guide for
caregivers / Maria M. Meyer and Paula Derr ; with
Jon Caswell.
    p. cm.
    Includes index.
    ISBN 0-9664767-8-6

    1. Home care services—Handbooks, manuals, etc.
2. Caregivers—Handbooks, manuals, etc. 3. Cerebrovascular
disease. I. Derr, Paula. II. Caswell, Jon.
III. Title.

RA645.3.M497 2007   649.8
                              QBI06-600542

Cover Art and Text Illustration: Stacey L. Tandberg
Interior Design: Frank Loose
Cover Design: David Kessler
Page Layout: International Graphic Services

Distributed to the Trade by Publishers Group West.
Printed in the United States of America.

07 08 09 10 11 / 10 9 8 7 6 5 4 3 2 1

About the Authors

Maria M. Meyer has been a long-time advocate of social causes, beginning with her work as co-founder of the Society for Abused Children of the Children's Home Society of Florida and founding executive director of the Children's Foundation of Greater Miami. When her father-in-law suffered a stroke in 1993, Maria became aware of the need for better information about how to care for an aging parent, a responsibility shared by millions of Americans. That experience led Maria to found CareTrust Publications and to co-author the award-winning guide, *The Comfort of Home™: An Illustrated Step-by-Step Guide for Caregivers*, earning the Benjamin Franklin Award in the health category. She is a keynote speaker and workshop leader on caregiver topics to health care professionals and community groups, as well as a Caregiver Community Action Network volunteer for the National Family Caregiver Association.

Paula Derr has been employed by the Sisters of Providence Health System for over 25 years and is clinical educator for three emergency departments in the Portland metropolitan area. She is co-owner of InforMed, which publishes emergency medical services field guides for emergency medical technicians (EMTs), paramedics, firefighters, physicians, and nurses and has co-authored numerous health care articles. For Paula, home care is a family tradition of long standing. For many years, Paula cared for her mother and grandmother in her home while raising two daughters and maintaining her career in nursing and health care management. Her personal and professional experience adds depth to many chapters of this book. Paula is active in several prominent professional organizations—SCCM, ENA, AACN, NFNA—and holds both local and national board positions. Paula is a native Oregonian and lives with her husband in Portland.

Jon Caswell has been lead editor and staff writer of *Stroke Connection Magazine*, published by the American Stroke Association, for more than 10 years. During that time he has written about many of the emotional travails and triumphs of stroke survivors and their caregivers. Over the years he has covered most of the scientific developments that are improving the lives of stroke families. In addition to his career as a writer, Jon was an instructor in the Wellness Department of Southern Methodist University for 15 years. He teaches "Finding Time Sitting Still," a meditation class, with Linda, his wife of 25 years. They live in Dallas, Texas.

Our Mission

CareTrust Publications is committed to providing high-quality, user-friendly information to those who face an illness or the responsibilities of caring for friends, family, or clients.

Dedication

For all those whose lives are forever touched by stroke.

Dear Caregiver,

Caring for someone with an illness like stroke can be deeply satisfying as well as uniquely challenging. Partners, family, and friends can be drawn more closely together when they meet these challenges. Yet, caregiving can also be physically and emotionally exhausting, especially for the person who is the primary caregiver.

The Comfort of Home™ for Stroke: A Guide for Caregivers offers basic yet complete answers to your questions about caregiving for a person with a stroke. Although the book discusses issues specific to caring for a stroke survivor, it also contains valuable information that will be of help to any caregiver. This guide to in-home care uses current best practices in the areas it covers. It offers practical tips for many activities of daily living and the more complicated and stressful situations a caregiver may face. It also includes a wide-ranging list of resources for further reading and study.

The *Guide* is divided into three parts:

Part One, Getting Ready, describes stroke and its causes and how to prepare for the task of caregiving to someone who has had a stroke. It shows how to set up a home in a safe and comfortable way for the person whose needs are changing and abilities are declining because of a stroke. Perhaps most important, it teaches you how to communicate better with doctors, nurses, aides, pharmacists and insurance companies to get the services you need.

Part Two, Day by Day, guides you through every aspect of daily care for the stroke survivor. This may be as basic as activities of daily living, such as bathing or helping someone transfer from a chair to a bed, or as daring as traveling abroad with a person whose health is declining or who is handicapped by a stroke.

Part Three, Additional Resources, provides a list of common medical abbreviations to help you understand the terms that many health care-professionals use. There is information about medical specialists who can be part of the health care team and a glossary of terms used to describe and explain symptoms or conditions.

Because a picture is worth a thousand words, we frequently use illustrations throughout the *Guide*. We also include information on organizations and publications that will be invaluable in helping you provide care.

Being a caregiver is not for the timid and fearful. However, having as much knowledge as possible will help you overcome your fears. With this guide in hand, you will understand what help is needed and learn where to find it or how to provide it yourself.

Warm regards,

Maria & Paula

Maria and Paula

Acknowledgments

The procedures described in this *Guide* are based on research and consultation with experts in the fields of stroke nursing, medicine, and design. The authors thank the innumerable professionals and caregivers who have assisted in the development of this book. We are especially grateful to the following reviewers who made comments on sections of the *Stroke* manuscript during its development. We thank them for their significant contributions, without which the quality and comprehensiveness of this *Guide* would not have been possible. Some sections of this volume are adapted from other editions in *The Comfort of Home*™ Series. We extend our gratitude to those authors and organizations whose contributions have enhanced this book.

Barry J. Jacobs, Psy.D.
Director of Behavioral Sciences
Crozer-Keystone Family Medicine Residency Program
Author, *The Emotional Survival Guide for Caregivers*

Cheryl L. Shigaki, Ph.D.
Assistant Professor
Department of Health Psychology
School of Health Professions
University of Missouri

Joan S. Grant, DSN, RN, CS
Professor
School of Nursing
University of Alabama at Birmingham

We are especially grateful to the following reviewers who made comments on sections of the *The Comfort of Home*™ during its development:

Judy Alleman, RN, MN
CNS, Gerontology,
Professor, Mental Health Nursing,
Clark College

Mary J. Amdall-Thompson, RN, MS
Program Executive-Professional Services,
Oregon Board of Nursing

Sonya Beebe, RN
Executive Director,
Elder Abode, Lincoln City, Oregon

Brad Bowman, MD
CEO, WellMed, Inc.

Beth Boyd-Roberts, PT
Physical Therapy–In-Patient
Supervisor

Karen Foley, OTR
Director, Regional Rehabilitation
Services

Ruth Freeman, CNA
Caregiver

Kay B. Girsberger, RD

Esther King, RN, MN
Professor of Nursing, Clark College

Toni Lonning, MSW, LCSW
Social Worker/Care Manager

Betty McCallum, RN, BSN

Sylvia McSkimming, PhD, RD
Executive Director,
Supportive Care of the Dying:
A Coalition for Compassionate Care

James L. Meyer, AIA

Donald E. Nielsen, AIA

Northwest Parish Nurses Board of
Directors

Cheryl Olson, RN, MBA
Director of Clinical Operations,
Home Services

Pamela Pauli, RN, MN

David L. Sanders, AIA
President, HPD Cambridge

Annette Stixrud, RN, MS
Program Director,
Northwest Parish Nurse Ministries

James Sturgis
Executive Director, Rose Villa, Inc.

Diane Welch, RN, MN
Associate Professor of Nursing,
Linfield College

We thank them for their significant contributions, without which the quality and comprehensiveness of this *Guide* would not have been possible.

To Our Readers

We believe *The Comfort of Home™ for Stroke: A Guide for Caregivers* reflects currently accepted practice in the areas it covers. However, the authors and publisher assume no liability with respect to the accuracy, completeness, or application of information presented here.

The Comfort of Home™ for Stroke is not meant to replace medical care but to add to the medical advice and services you receive from health care professionals. You should seek professional medical advice from a health care provider. This book is only a guide; follow your common sense and good judgment.

Neither the authors nor the publisher are engaged in rendering legal, accounting, or other professional advice. Seek the services of a competent professional if legal, architectural, or other expert assistance is required. The *Guide* does not represent Americans with Disabilities Act compliance.

Every effort has been made at the time of publication to provide accurate names, addresses, and phone numbers in the resource sections at the ends of chapters. The resources listed are those that benefit readers nationally. For this reason we have not included many local groups that offer valuable assistance. Failure to include an organization does not mean that it does not provide a valuable service. On the other hand, inclusion does not imply an endorsement. The authors and publisher do not warrant or guarantee any of the products described in this book and did not perform any independent analysis of the products described.

Throughout the book, we use "he" and "she" interchangeably when referring to the caregiver and the person being cared for.

ATTENTION NONPROFIT ORGANIZATIONS, CORPORATIONS, AND PROFESSIONAL ORGANIZATIONS: *The Comfort of Home™ Stroke Edition* is available at special quantity discounts for bulk purchases for gifts, fundraising, or educational training purposes. Special books, book excerpts, or booklets can also be created to fit specific needs. For details, write to CareTrust Publications LLC, P.O. Box 10283, Portland, Oregon 97296-0283, or call 1-800-565-1533.

CONTENTS AT A GLANCE

Praise for *The Comfort of Home*™ Caregiver Guides

"This is an invaluable addition to bibliographies for the home caregiver. Hospital libraries will want to have a copy on hand for physicians, nurses, social workers, chaplains, and any staff dealing with MS patients and their caregivers. Highly recommended for all public libraries and consumer health collections."
—*Library Journal*

"A well-organized format with critical information and resources at your finger-tips . . . educates the reader about the many issues that stand before people living with chronic conditions and provides answers and avenues for getting the best care possible."
—MSWorld, Inc. www.msworld.org

"A masterful job of presenting the multiple aspects of caregiving in a format that is both comprehensive and reader-friendly . . . important focus on physical aspects of giving care."
—Parkinson Report

"Almost any issue or question or need for resolution is most likely spoken of somewhere within the pages of this guide."
—*American Journal of Alzheimer's Disease*

"Physicians, family practitioners and geriatricians, and hospital social workers should be familiar with the book and recommend it to families of the elderly."
—Reviewers Choice, Home Care University

"An excellent guide on caregiving in the home. Home health professionals will find it to be a useful tool in teaching family caregivers."
—Five Star Rating, *Doody's Health Sciences Review Journal*

"Overall a beautifully designed book with very useful, practical information for caregivers."
—Judges from the Benjamin Franklin Awards

"Noteable here are the specifics. Where others focus on psychology alone, this gets down to the nitty gritty."
—*The Midwest Book Review*

"We use *The Comfort of Home*™ for the foundational text in our 40-hour Caregiver training. I believe it is the best on the market."
—Linda Young, Project Manager, College of the Desert

Part One: Getting Ready

Chapter

Understanding Stroke—One Disease, Two Causes

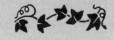

Understanding Stroke— One Disease, Two Causes

When a family member survives a stroke, that event affects everyone in the family, most of all the caregiver. The effects begin immediately. Unlike gradually worsening diseases, such as Alzheimer's disease, where family members take on more responsibilities with time, stroke caregivers are put into that role almost overnight. One day you're leading a normal life, and then the person in your care has a stroke, and suddenly another person is dependent on you, possibly for everything from eating to bathing to toileting.

In addition to the physical changes it brings, stroke often alters cognitive (thinking) ability, speech, and emotions. Not to mention that any or all of these changes vary in appearance or intensity, so no one can really tell you how best to approach your situation.

Overnight, you may have been thrown into a full-time job you did not ask for, were not trained for, and that has no end date. When put into this situation, you may feel guilt, anger, fear, that you are unable to do the job, that you are a victim, as well as continuous stress. In order to survive, you will have to set limits and you will have to enforce rules, neither of which is comfortable. If you don't set limits and enforce rules, however, your life will become unmanageable, and the person you're caring for will suffer.

It is very important that you know from the beginning that you have to find ways to take care of yourself. This self-care is not an indulgence, it is a necessity, and you have to make it happen. Maybe you fit a walk in while the person in your care is napping, or do 10 minutes of yoga after he has gone to bed, or you might read a book before he wakes up. Whatever you do, do something every day, even if it's just a little bit.

Here's why *every day* is so important: Stress is cumulative. It grows. You can't take stress away from caregiving, but you can reduce it. To do so you have to take care of yourself in some way each day. Think of this time—walking, reading, bathing, meditating, whatever you choose—as a pause in your day where you can feel free—if just for a few minutes. Decide now that you will do this for yourself. It will make a big difference in how you feel.

One of the best things you can do for yourself and for the person you are helping is to find a stroke support group—many have separate caregiver groups. These groups are wonderful places to get help and information for both of you. Not only is the group a place to talk about your feelings, but it is also a place to get real-world answers to problems from people who have been there. They know exactly what you are going through.

 To find a support group in your area, log on to the American Stroke Association (ASA) Web site, www.Stroke Association.org/strokegroup and enter your ZIP code. If you don't have access to the Internet, call the ASA Warmline 1-888-4-STROKE (478-7653). In addition, churches and community centers sometimes sponsor caregiver-only support groups. If there's nothing like this in your area, start one yourself. The ASA has information on that as well.

When you contact the ASA, subscribe to *Stroke Connection Magazine*. It's free and will give you helpful information and stories of inspiration.

> **NOTE** How we speak of ourselves is how we think of ourselves. It is important to use supportive, positive words. The terms "stroke survivor" and "stroke victim" are an example. "Stroke victim" makes a person feel weak and ill, while "stroke survivor" gives the person the strength and courage to move on. Surviving a stroke and working at recovery require strength of body and spirit. For that reason, stroke patients will be called "survivors" in this book.

Understanding Stroke—One Disease, Two Causes

Here is an easy way to understand how a stroke happens. Stroke is one disease with two causes and many consequences. The kind of stroke a person has is decided by what the stroke does to a person's arteries (vessels that carry blood from the heart through the body)—they are either blocked (ischemic) or broken (hemorrhagic).

Blocked Artery Stroke (Ischemic)

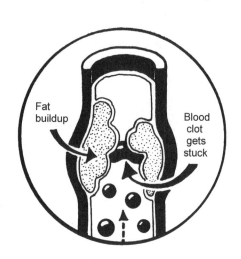

Fat buildup

Blood clot gets stuck

An *ischemic* (pronounced is-kemik) stroke is caused by a clot that blocks an artery in the brain or leading to the brain. This clot stops or slows the blood flow and starves the brain cells of oxygen and they die. The blockage may be the result of a blood clot formed in the heart because of a heart problem, or it may be a piece of plaque that has broken off from hardening of the arteries (an atherosclerotic deposit in a blood vessel). Whatever the cause of the blockage, the longer the brain goes without blood, the greater the damage—a modern medical saying is "**time lost is brain lost**." Ischemic (blocked artery) stroke accounts for about 9 out of 10 strokes.

Broken Artery Stroke (Hemorrhagic)

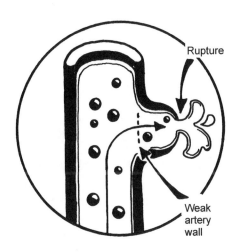

Rupture

Weak artery wall

The second type of stroke is caused by a burst blood vessel (*hemorrhagic*; pronounced hem-a-rajik) that leaks blood into the brain. The bleeding irritates the piece of the brain it touches and causes swelling, which in turn damages the brain. There are many reasons vessels break, but high blood pressure is the most common.

There are two types of broken artery strokes—

1. bleeding inside the brain (intracerebral hemorrhage)

2. bleeding into the area between the brain and skull (subarachnoid hemorrhage)

Although only 12 percent of strokes are the broken-artery kind (hemorrhagic), they are more deadly.

NOTE Close to 40 percent of bleeding strokes result in death within a month compared to about 10 percent of blockage strokes.

Mini-strokes (TIAs)

In addition to these types of strokes, there are mini-strokes, which are officially called "TIAs" or "transient ischemic accidents." A TIA is a stroke in every way except for the length of time it lasts and the damage it causes. In other words, the clot moves in some way and blood flow is restored. As a caregiver, you should know that people who have TIAs are more likely to have an actual stroke, but most strokes come as a surprise and do not follow a TIA. The important thing to remember is that if your survivor reports any stroke symptoms listed as warning signs (see *Stroke Warning Signs*, p. 14), it is a medical emergency, **dial 9-1-1**. Remember, **time lost is brain lost**.

see *Stroke Warning Signs*, p. 14

> **NOTE** Stroke is the third leading cause of death after heart disease and all types of cancer, and it is a leading cause of disability.

Endless Consequences

There may only be two causes (blocked or broken artery) of stroke, but the kinds of things that happen to a person when brain cells die from the bleeding in the brain have a huge effect on the survivor's life. *Every* stroke is different. The changes in ability that survivors face after a stroke are called "deficits." The deficits that a stroke leaves behind are decided by which brain cells are killed, not how they were killed.

Stroke deficits can go from mild speech impairment or muscle weakness to "locked-in syndrome," where survivors are completely conscious (awake) but cannot move anything but their eyes. Stroke may result in paralysis (muscles can't move), cognitive (brain) damage, or uncontrollable emotions. It can be all of those things or none, for there are still many other possibilities, such as double vision or the inability to swallow, read, or speak at all. A survivor can lose the ability to remember faces or remember anything at all.

Tip Just as a car never works the same after an accident, a stroke survivor's body and mind don't work the same after the stroke. The changes in mind and body the survivor faces are his "deficits."

Deficits (Losses) and the Brain

The part of the brain that is damaged will determine how a person is affected by a stroke. Remember that if a stroke occurs on the left side of the brain, it is the right side of the body that is affected; if the stroke occurs on the right side of the brain, it is the left side of the body that is affected.

Right Side (Hemisphere)

Some of the major functions (jobs) of the right side of the brain include perception (the ability to take in and understand information) and control of the *left* side of the body. A stroke affecting this side can cause changes like these:

- inability to judge distances, which can cause falls

- loss of hand–eye coordination

- loss of short-term memory

- neglecting or ignoring anything on the left of the body (left-side neglect)

- poor impulse control (can't keep yourself from doing something you probably shouldn't do) and loss of control over emotions (emotional lability, reflex or sudden crying or laughing)

- left-side paralysis (*left hemiplegia*; pronounced hem-a plee-ja)

- left-side weakness (*left hemiparesis*; pronounced hem-a-pa-ree-sus)

Left Side (Hemisphere)

Some of the major functions (jobs) of the left side of the brain include speech and control of the *right* side of the body. A stroke affecting the left side can cause many changes, including—

- right-side paralysis (right hemiplegia)

- right-side weakness (right hemiparesis)

- various problems with speech and communication (*aphasia*; pronounced a-fa-zha, *apraxia*; pronounced a-prak-sia)

- short-term memory loss

Cerebellum

Some of the major functions of the *cerebellum* (the large, back part of the brain; pronounced ser-a-bell-um) include coordination and balance. A stroke affecting the cerebellum can cause many changes, including—

- dizziness

- nausea and vomiting

- loss of coordination

- a tendency to lose balance and fall

- slurred speech

Brain Stem

The major jobs of the brain stem are controlling breathing, heart rate, and blood pressure. A stroke affecting the brain stem can cause many changes, including—

- complete paralysis ("locked-in syndrome")

- coma

- double vision

- swallowing difficulties

- death

What's Left After the Stroke?

There is no way to predict what deficits (losses) a survivor will be left with, how severe those deficits will be, or how long they will last. Most doctors claim that whatever the survivor has regained in the first six months to a year is what she will be left with forever.

 If you go to a stroke support group, you will hear personal stories to disprove the six-month rule. The biggest gains may come in the first few months, but smaller changes often occur as a result of repeated effort over a much longer period of time. Even when official rehab stops, it is to your benefit to find ways for your survivor to be as active as possible.

Recovery has a lot to do with the survivor wanting to get better and the need to keep working at it, and you as caregiver can help with encouragement and emotional support. The more the survivor can do on her own, the better she will feel about herself and the freer you will be. It is your job and it also helps you if you let the survivor do whatever she can for herself, even though it may take longer.

Tip If you do not encourage your survivor to be independent, then he will depend more on you. Your goal is for him to be as independent as his deficits allow while remaining safe.

Living in the Plateaus

People recovering from stroke may come to a point where they cannot improve anymore in their physical recovery, this is called hitting a plateau. But even when a person is no longer increasing grip strength or improving speech, he or she can continue to recover emotionally.

> **NOTE** There is an important point in this process of emotional recovery. It occurs when the person who has had a stroke stops seeing herself as a victim and realizes that she is a survivor. As one support group leader said, *"There are no 'victims' in this room. All the stroke 'victims' are dead."*

Stroke Survivor Depression Is Common

It is natural for any person who has had a trauma to be depressed. But because stroke is a brain injury, it may also change brain chemistry and cause "organic" (coming from the body itself) depression. There is also depression that arises from the situation of having your life changed so very much, perhaps permanently. Do not allow depression to go untreated because it limits your survivor's recovery and puts his or her independence at risk. We will talk about *caregiver* depression later. (See *Negative Emotions That May Arise in You*, p. 166.)

Symptoms of Depression

Some of the symptoms of depression include—

- long-lasting sad, anxious, or "empty" mood
- feelings of hopelessness, pessimism
- feelings of guilt, worthlessness, helplessness
- loss of interest or pleasure in hobbies and activities that were once enjoyed, including sex
- decreased energy, always feeling tired, being "slowed down"

- difficulty concentrating, remembering, making decisions

- insomnia, early-morning awakening, or oversleeping

- appetite and/or weight changes

- thoughts of death or suicide, or suicidal attempts

- restlessness, irritability

If five or more of these symptoms last for longer than two weeks, depression may be the cause. Talk to your physician or psychiatrist about treatment options. The most effective treatment combines medication with talking therapy.

Not only does depression influence the speed (rate) of the survivor's physical recovery, it is also a risk factor in having a second stroke and even cardiovascular disease.

Identifying Stroke

There are definite stroke warning signs. You may not have known them before the stroke of the person in your care, but it is time to learn them now, for two reasons:

- First, having had a stroke, **your survivor is at increased risk of another stroke.** Almost a third of the estimated 700,000 strokes that occur each year in the United States are "recurrent" strokes. The risk of another stroke among stroke and TIA survivors is as high as 40 percent within five years.

- Second, if your survivor is a blood relative, then his or her stroke means *your* risk is increased. The Framingham Study shows that a parent's stroke before age 65 meant that their children had three times the risk of having a stroke by age 65.

Stroke is a medical emergency. Know these warning signs and teach them to others in your family. Every second counts.

Stroke Warning Signs

If a person is having a stroke, he may have one or more of these symptoms—

- sudden numbness or weakness of the face, arm, or leg, especially on one side of the body

- sudden confusion, trouble speaking, or understanding

- sudden trouble seeing in one or both eyes

- sudden trouble walking, dizziness, loss of balance or coordination

- sudden, severe headache with no known cause

If you see that the person in your care has any one of these symptoms, it is a medical emergency. **Call 9-1-1 immediately!** Don't wait to see if the symptom goes away. Don't wait to see if the symptom gets worse or if other symptoms develop. **Time lost is brain lost!**

Why Quick Response Is Critical

Because brain cells die very quickly after a stroke begins, it is urgent to get treatment as soon as possible. If a stroke is left to run its course, millions of brain cells will die. Prompt treatment can stop that.

At this time there is one FDA-approved drug for the treatment of acute blocked artery (*ischemic*) stroke. However, this drug, called tPA, *can only be used within three hours of the start of symptoms.* Most people go to the ER long after that treatment window has passed and so are not able to take tPA. Because of this, fewer than 2 percent of blockage (ischemic) stroke patients currently receive this potentially life-saving treatment.

What Is tPA Medication?

tPA stands for "tissue plasminogen activator." It is a super clot-buster introduced into the patient's bloodstream. It dissolves the clot that is blocking blood flow, therefore, it can only be used in blockage strokes. This requires that the patient undergo some type of imaging, either an MRI or CT scan, (a special type of X ray that allows doctors to see the body parts very clearly) to be sure that the type of stroke the person is having is a blockage (ischemic) stroke, rather than a broken-artery stroke. Using tPA in a broken-artery (hemorrhagic) stroke would be fatal.

The three-hour window cannot be extended and even includes the time needed for the image scan. tPA has resulted in symptoms being lessened and even reversed, but most patients do not arrive at the hospital in time for it to be used. If it is not known when symptoms began, doctors won't even consider using tPA.

There are several new drugs under consideration for the treatment of acute (sudden) stroke. Some of these drugs will lengthen the three-hour treatment window, but at this time, only tPA medication is used. Even when new drugs become available, this medical truth will remain—**Time lost is brain lost!** No drug will bring dead brain cells back to life.

Tip Not all hospitals have tPA medication. It is only available at larger hospitals and those designated as "primary stroke centers." Studies indicate that patients who go to primary stroke centers have better outcomes. Because your survivor is at increased risk, it would be a good idea for you to identify hospitals in your area that have received stroke-center certification from the Joint Commission on the Accreditation of Healthcare Organizations (JCAHO). Go to www.jcaho.org and click the "Certification Programs" tab, then click "Primary Stroke Centers."

A Quick Way to Diagnose Stroke—FAST

Many emergency technicians (EMTs) use the Cincinnati Stroke Scale to diagnose stroke in the people they are helping. Working off the acronym (a word made from the first letters of a phrase) FAST, this scale shows quickly if a person has had a stroke.

Cincinnati Stroke Scale

Cincinnati Stroke Scale
(check if abnormal)

❏ **F (face)** FACIAL DROOP: Have patient smile or show teeth. Is the smile even or lop-sided?

Normal: Both sides of the face move equally or not at all.

Abnormal: One side of the patient's face droops.

❏ **A (arm)** MOTOR WEAKNESS: Arm drift (patient closes eyes, extends arms, palms up)

Normal: Arms remain extended equally, or move equally or do not move at all.

Abnormal: One arm drops down when compared with the other.

❏ **S (speech)** "You can't teach an old dog new tricks." (repeat phrase)

Normal: Phrase is repeated clearly and correctly.

Abnormal: Words are slurred (dysarthria) or abnormal (aphasia), or he can't speak.

❏ **T (time)** TIME LAST SEEN NORMAL: ____

The FAST test has proven to be very good at predicting stroke, and not just for emergency medical technicians (EMTs). Like knowing the warning signs, it is another helpful tool that stroke caregivers and families can use to reduce the time to treatment.

Stroke Often Changes Personality

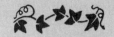

Stroke Often Changes Personality

*O*f all the areas of life that stroke affects, its impact on the survivor's personality may be the most difficult for family and friends to understand and get used to. Emotional changes are typical after any type of stroke. Depression is very common after any life-changing health challenge, especially if it results in a loss of independence. (See **Stroke Survivor Depression Is Common**, p. 12.)

Although depression is the most common emotional change after stroke, other psychological or mental changes can make the survivor feel upset or frustrated.

Cognitive Challenges

Cognitive deficits are changes in thinking, like having trouble solving problems. This category also includes dementia and memory problems, as well as many kinds of communication challenges.

 Tip Short-term memory problems tend to show up in people with left-brain stroke. This may make it difficult for them to learn new information. Expect to repeat things and remind your survivor of things over and over.

Right-brain strokes cause different kinds of memory problems—these survivors have the tendency to get things out of sequence (when asked to get dressed the survivor might put on his shoes, then put on his socks) or to misunderstand or confuse information.

- These survivors may mix up the details surrounding an event.

- They might recall events but get confused about *when* they happened or *who* was involved.

- They might think someone had visited in the morning rather than at night.

Communication in all its forms often changes after a stroke, but where the stroke occurred in the brain makes a difference as to what will be affected. In addition to communication problems like aphasia, a condition affecting the ability to understand language, communication deficits may include decreased attention, an inability to keep focused on something (distractibility), and the inability to inhibit behavior that is not right for the situation. (For more on aphasia, see *Communication Changes After Stroke*, p. 244.)

Tip

Some survivors lose the ability to *read* people, for instance, they can't understand the emotional meaning of a message or understand body language. Some have a deficit called *perseveration,* which means the person is unable to stop himself from doing things. Survivors with this deficit can't seem to "put the brakes on," for instance, they can't get off a specific topic during conversation. This can be extremely difficult for family members.

Problem-solving ability is sometimes affected, usually more in survivors of right-brain strokes. This may be due in part to right-brain survivors being more impulsive and less aware of their deficits. They think they can do things safely that they actually can't do, like getting up and walking or driving. They fail to think before they act. They aren't thinking through situations.

What Can Be Done

Cognitive rehabilitation helps survivors learn to think in sequence again or provides new behavior to overcome this problem. Cognitive rehabilitation is usually provided by speech therapists. Neuropsychologists (doctors who combine an understanding of behavior with the way the brain and nervous system work) and occupational therapists can also help with cognitive rehab. There are computer software programs available to help survivors regain skills, but check with a therapist before making a purchase.

Survivors can use a notebook to write down important information to jog their memory; PDAs (personal digital assistants) are also useful for this purpose. Computer games and activities to exercise the mind—like word puzzles, *Wheel of Fortune*, playing cards, or dominoes are also helpful. A grandchild might be a perfect game-mate.

Personality Changes

Some survivors don't seem to care about anything (apathy). It is easy to mistake apathy for depression because the person is content to sit and stare at the wall all day.

NOTE The difference between apathy and depression is that with apathy the person seems not to have emotions or to care about anything. People with apathy are not motivated or interested in things. They are generally satisfied and content with doing nothing. This is seen more often in right-brain strokes.

Depression, on the other hand, is an emotion in which the person feels sad and often discouraged, hopeless about the future, perhaps even says he wants to kill himself. The person does not feel content or satisfied. Depression is common in both left- and right-brain strokes.

What You Can Do

Whether apathetic or depressed, the best response is to get your survivor active and moving. Give her a choice of what to do or where to go, but make it clear she must choose to do something. Lying in bed all day or staying in her pajamas is not an option.

Neglect

Right-brain survivors may experience what is called "neglect." Neglect is an attentional disorder in which the stroke survivor does not pay attention to or notice things on one side of the body. Neglect can range from someone who doesn't recognize paralyzed limbs as his own to someone who ignores food on one side of the plate, or words on one side of the page.

> **NOTE** Driving is extremely dangerous for anyone with neglect.

What You Can Do

Family members can help survivors who have neglect by encouraging them to pay attention to the neglected side. Talking to them from that side helps them to focus and concentrate on that side. It also helps to put the phone on that side or touch that side of the body when you talk to them. Stimulating the neglected side and encouraging the survivor to use it helps the person use that side.

Impulsiveness

Another personality change that occurs after stroke is impulsiveness. Survivors with this disorder don't think ahead. They may move too quickly, or try to drive when they have left-side neglect. This is seen more in people with right-side or frontal lobe strokes.

What You Can Do

There are things you can do to help with impulsiveness (acting suddenly without considering the consequences), for example, hide the car keys. You can remind the survivor to slow down or put a lap belt on a chair so he or she can't just jump up. Consistent verbal and visual cuing (a finger held up to the lips is a visual cue to be quiet) and repeated reminders can help a person with poor impulse control to slow down.

 Tip Always treat the person with respect and listen to his side of the story.

Here are some hints for helping a stroke survivor who may be demonstrating inappropriate or unsafe behaviors—

1. Offer praise when the person is exhibiting safe, appropriate, or correct behaviors ("*You really handled that situation well, I'm so glad you decided to take the bus rather than drive...*")

2. Allow the person to choose among appropriate and safe choices ("*Do you want me to drive you, or would you rather take a cab?*")

3. Be firm and set necessary limits. Explain your concerns and feelings in a supportive way ("*I know you want to use your power tools, but I care too much about you to let you use them at this time.*")

Are These Changes Permanent?

Personality changes after stroke are intense for both survivors and family members, and there is no guarantee that they will go away. Sometimes people mellow out, sometimes they don't.

Certainly, depression need not be permanent, especially with the many choices of anti-depressant drugs and the increasing availability of talk therapy and support groups.

NOTE A lot of emotional healing requires active social support. Isolation may feel like the easiest response, but it is not healthy for *you*, the caregiver, or *your survivor*. There is life after stroke, but you have to stay active and stay around people. Support groups are crucial for stroke recovery. For help in finding a support group near you, call the American Stroke Association Warmline, 1-888-4-STROKE (478-7653) or visit www.StrokeAssociation.org/strokegroup and enter your ZIP code.

Stroke Risk Factors

Stroke Risk Factors

*R*isk factors are traits and lifestyle habits that increase the chance of disease. A lot of studies have identified several factors that increase the risk of stroke. There are two groups of stroke risk factors—

- those that you can *change, control, or treat*
- those that can't *be changed.*

The more risk factors, the greater the chance of having a stroke. The best way to prevent a stroke is to reduce the stroke risk factors. A doctor can help you change factors that result from lifestyle or environment.

> **NOTE** Stroke **risk factors** predispose a person to stroke. They are not **symptoms** of a stroke. It is possible to have risk factors without having a stroke.
>
> Stroke **warning signs** are symptoms of a stroke. If you are experiencing a warning sign, you are having a stroke or TIA. It is not possible to have a warning sign without having a stroke. (Review the warning signs at the beginning of the book, see p. 14.)

Controllable Risk Factors

Lifestyle changes may affect some of these risk factors, however, when lifestyle changes don't reduce the risk factor enough, get medical help to control it.

- **High blood pressure**—High blood pressure (140/90 mm Hg or higher) is the most important risk factor for stroke. It usually has no specific symptoms and no early warning signs. Get your survivor's and *your* blood pressure checked regularly.

NOTE

Use a blood pressure cuff to monitor blood pressure at home. It's simple to use and gives a much better picture of your survivor's blood pressure situation than irregular trips to the doctor.

Two-thirds of those who have first strokes have blood pressure higher than 160/95. Those with these numbers have *four times* the risk of stroke as someone with normal blood pressure.

- **Smoking**—Cigarette smoking is a major, preventable risk factor for stroke. The nicotine and carbon monoxide in tobacco smoke reduce the oxygen in a person's blood. They also damage the walls of blood vessels and make clots more likely to form. Some kinds of birth control pills combined with smoking greatly increase stroke risk in women. *If you or your survivor smoke, get help to quit NOW!*

NOTE

The relative risk of stroke in heavy smokers (more than 40 cigarettes a day) is twice that of people who smoke fewer than 10 cigarettes a day. Stroke risk decreases significantly after two years of not smoking and is at the level of non-smokers within five years of quitting.

- **Diabetes**—Diabetes is defined as a fasting (tested on an empty stomach) blood sugar level of 126 mg/dL or more measured on two occasions. Even when diabetes is treated, having it still increases stroke risk. Many people with diabetes also have high blood pressure, high blood cholesterol, and are overweight, increasing their risk even more. If you or your survivor have diabetes, work closely with your doctor to manage it.

- **Carotid or other artery disease**—The carotid arteries in your neck supply blood to your brain. If these arteries become narrowed by fatty deposits (called "plaque") from atherosclerosis, they may become blocked by a blood clot. PAD (peripheral artery disease) is the narrowing of blood vessels carrying blood to leg and arm muscles. People with PAD have a higher risk of carotid artery disease and an increased risk of stroke.

- **Atrial fibrillation (a-fib)**—This is a heart rhythm disorder where the heart's upper chambers (atria) quiver instead of contracting effectively. Because of this, blood can pool and form clots. If a clot enters the bloodstream and lodges in an artery leading to or in the brain, a stroke results.

- **Other heart disease**—People with coronary heart disease or heart failure have a higher risk of stroke than those with hearts that work normally. An enlarged heart, heart valve disease, and some types of congenital heart defects also increase stroke risk.

- **"TIAs" (transient ischemic attacks)**—TIAs are "mini-strokes" caused by blood vessel blockage that becomes unclogged on its own and produces no lasting damage. Think of TIAs as "warning strokes." However, most strokes are not preceded by TIAs. Stroke and TIA have exactly the same warning signs. If you see any of them, it is a medical emergency, dial 9-1-1.

- **Certain blood disorders**—A high red blood cell count thickens the blood and makes clots more likely. Doctors may treat this problem by removing blood cells or prescribing "blood thinners." *Sickle cell disease* (also called sickle cell anemia) is a genetic (family history) disorder that mainly affects African Americans and makes red blood cells less capable of carrying oxygen.

They also tend to stick to vessel walls, which can block arteries to the brain and cause a stroke.

- **High blood cholesterol**—A high level of total cholesterol (240 mg/dL or higher) is a major risk factor for heart disease, which raises stroke risk. High levels of *LDL (less desirable; lousy or bad) cholesterol* (greater than 100 mg/dL) and *triglycerides* (blood fats, 150 mg/dL or higher) increase the risk of stroke in people with previous coronary heart disease, ischemic stroke, or TIA. Low levels (less than 40 mg/dL for men; less than 50 mg/dL for women) of *HDL (highly desirable; healthy or good) cholesterol* also may raise stroke risk. (📖 For more on cholesterol, see *Diet, Nutrition, and Exercise*, p. 264.)

NOTE ▷ Hardening of the arteries (atherosclerosis) is the process in which deposits of fatty substances, cholesterol, cellular waste products, calcium, and other substances build up in the inner lining of an artery. This buildup is called "plaque."

Everybody has atherosclerosis, even young children. The only variable (difference) is how much atherosclerosis a person has. It starts in the aorta (main arterial trunk that carries blood from the heart to the arteries for distribution throughout the body) and progressively narrows arteries and makes them less flexible, decreasing blood flow, and increasing blood pressure.

- **Physical inactivity and obesity**—Inactivity and obesity both can increase the risk of high blood pressure, high blood cholesterol, diabetes, heart disease, and stroke. Depending on his deficits, exercise may be difficult for your survivor, nonetheless, it is very important. Find a way he can be active. (📖 See *Diet, Nutrition, and Exercise*, p. 272. See *Range of Motion*, p. 235.)

- **Excessive alcohol**—Women who drink on average more than one alcoholic drink a day or men who drink more than two drinks a day can raise blood pressure and may increase their stroke risk.

- **Some illegal drugs**—Intravenous drug abuse carries a high risk of stroke. Cocaine use has also been linked to strokes and heart attacks.

Risk factors you *can't* modify—

- **Increasing age**—People of all ages, including children, have strokes. However, roughly two-thirds of all strokes occur in people over age 65. Stroke risk doubles in each succeeding decade, so a 75-year-old has twice the risk of a 65-year-old.

- **Sex (gender)**—In most age groups, more men than women will have strokes in a given year. However, women account for more than half of all stroke deaths because they tend to have strokes later in life. Pregnant women have a higher stroke risk, as do women taking birth control pills who also smoke or have high blood pressure or other risk factors.

- **Heredity (family history)**—Blood relatives of people who have had strokes are at increased risk.

- **Race**—The risk of stroke among African Americans is twice that of Caucasians. This may be due to the fact that blacks have higher rates of high blood pressure, diabetes, and obesity. Increased rates of poverty and poor access to health care may also contribute.

NOTE In the eleven states of the so-called Stroke Belt, stroke rates are higher than in the rest of the country. Both blacks and whites in these states are at increased risk, but it is particularly high for African Americans. Basically, the Stroke Belt consists of the states of the Confederacy.

The states of North Carolina, South Carolina, and Georgia make up the "Stroke Buckle." Blacks and whites in these states have even higher stroke rates than the other states. African Americans in these states have among the highest stroke rates of any group anywhere in the world. Where the average age of first stroke is 65 for a white man in Minnesota, it is 45 for a black man in the Stroke Buckle.

- **Prior stroke or heart attack**—Anyone who has had a stroke is at much higher risk of having another one. About 28 percent of strokes happen in people who have already had one. Previous heart attacks also increase stroke risk.

What You Can (and Can't) Do

The first step in reducing your survivor's and your stroke risk is easy—assess that risk. Apply the list of risk factors to yourself and your survivor. Your survivor already has at least one risk factor that cannot be changed. If you find that you have risk factors that can't be modified, then start modifying all the risk factors you can. Implement a diet, exercise, and weight-loss program now. (📖 For more on post-stroke exercise, see *Diet, Nutrition, and Exercise*, p. 273.)

NOTE Check with a doctor before starting an exercise program, especially if you've been inactive for a long time.

Medication

It is quite likely that your survivor will leave the hospital with a hypertension (high blood pressure) prescription. Fill it immediately and be vigilant that the person in your care takes it *exactly* as directed.

At first, you will have to make medication management a priority. After awhile, it will become a habit.

> **NOTE** More than half of all prescriptions are taken incorrectly or not at all. No drug can work as expected if it's not taken as directed. High blood pressure medication must be taken as directed and NOT just when someone has symptoms.

Blood Pressure

Monitor your survivor's and your own blood pressure. If you have high blood pressure—and that would *not* be uncommon—and diet, exercise, and weight loss don't reduce it, then use medication prescribed by a doctor.

> **NOTE** High blood pressure is very bad for the cardiovascular system (heart and blood vessels). It makes the heart work harder, which makes the heart and blood vessels more prone to injury. Hypertension increases the risk of heart attack, stroke, congestive heart failure, atherosclerosis, and kidney failure. It damages the inner lining of arteries, which promotes the formation of plaque, which increases the risk of clots and narrows and hardens arteries, making them less elastic, which further increases blood pressure.

Cholesterol

Get both your survivor's and your cholesterol checked. High numbers may be changed by diet, exercise, and weight loss. If that doesn't work, check with the doctor about cholesterol-lowering drugs.

Diabetes

Get your survivor and yourself tested for diabetes and alter your lifestyle accordingly.

Depression

Depression is increasingly recognized as a risk factor for cardiovascular disease, including stroke. Check the list of symptoms on p. 12 and check with a doctor if you or your survivor have symptoms.

For reliable guidance in making healthy lifestyle changes, visit the Web site of the American Heart Association, www.HeartAssociation.org.

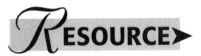

RESOURCE

The American Stroke Association
7272 Greenville Ave.
Dallas, TX 75231
www.StrokeAssociation.org
Stroke Family "Warmline"
(888) 4-STROKE (478-7653)

Is Home Care For You?

Is Home Care for You?

The need to provide care for another person arises for many reasons. Often, the person who needs care does not realize it and family members must step in to help make decisions. One of those decisions involves who the caregiver will be and where care will be provided. The choices can be difficult unless you know what to consider.

When one member of the family becomes disabled, roles within the family often change. A person who took care of the family in the past or was the income provider may become dependent, while another person in the family takes on added, often unfamiliar responsibilities. For a single person, the changes may involve a new dependence on non-family members. Just the word "dependence" can cause unpleasant feelings. Being able to talk openly about fears, anxiety, frustration, and doubts can be very helpful in dealing well with these new facts of life.

Discuss chronic care needs with the person's medical team to learn what treatments, adjustments and other changes may be necessary (see chapter 3). For some people, training to provide medical treatments and some long-range financial planning will be enough. For others, in-home personal assistance is the best option. Sometimes a nursing home or assisted living center is the better choice for everyone involved.

In making the decision for home care, it is important to be realistic about what your survivor needs, and what you, the caregiver, can provide in terms of time, kinds of care, and financial responsibility. For example, deciding to hire an in-home attendant may be necessary if the primary caregiver works full time. Before this happens, it's important to look at the financial and emotional issues that go along with this decision.

First, caregivers need to think about important issues such as independence, privacy, and the financial effect of hiring in-home help. Then the caregiver needs to talk to the survivor and others living in the home about these issues. How will the family pay for in-home help and how will it find the right person(s) or agency?

Before a person can be hired, the family needs to look at what kind of care is needed: **medical** *(symptom management, occupational or physical therapies, etc.),* **personal care** *(bathing, dressing, using the bathroom, etc.),* **homemaking** *(shopping, errands, laundry, housecleaning), or* **companionship** *(social outlets, safety issues, etc.).*

Your Support System

Sometimes children take on major household and personal care duties when a parent has disability. While it is positive for children to take on household jobs and tasks, their needs must be carefully balanced with the amount and level of caregiving they are expected to provide. Children are not equipped to handle the stress of being the main or primary caregiver. They should never be in charge of a parent's medical treatments or daily functions such as helping with the bathroom.

Family and friends can help. The first step is to let friends and family know that their help is needed and welcomed. Friends often worry that offering help might seem like meddling, especially when things seem to be going well.

Knowing What Level of Care Is Needed

Before you take on the demanding job of home care, decide what level of care you must provide. Do you need to give:

- minimum assistance?

- moderate assistance?

- maximum assistance?

In order to decide what level of care is needed, you must understand the person's condition and needs in the areas of daily care and health. Generally, these needs fall into two broad groups:

Activities of Daily Living (ADLs) such as eating, bathing, dressing, taking medicine, and going to the toilet.

Instrumental Activities of Daily Living (IADLs) are activities that are important to independence, such as cooking, shopping, housekeeping, getting to the doctor, paying bills, and managing money.

Things to look for in deciding the overall level of care needed are the person's—

- ability to get from bed to wheelchair without help

- ability to move without help in wheelchair or walker

- ability to manage bladder and bowel

- ability to carry out the basic activities of daily living

- ability to call for help

- degree of sight and hearing impairment

- degree of confusion

Also, consider emotional conditions that might require advanced or special levels of care:

- depression

- a need to be with other people or to have privacy

- homesickness

After giving some thought to the level of care that might be needed and the person's condition, abilities, and emotional state, try to place the person you might care for in one of these categories:

Minimum Assistance—This person is basically independent, can handle most household chores and personal care, and needs help with only one or two activities of daily living.

Moderate Assistance—This person needs help with three or more activities of daily living, such as bathing, cooking, or shopping.

Maximum Assistance—This person is unable to care for himself or herself, requires total assistance, and must be placed in a nursing home if no skilled caregiver is available in the home. Care is often provided by professionals, either in the home through home service agencies or in foster care homes, assisted living facilities, or nursing homes. At this level, serious problems are a real possibility.

Deciding Whether Home Care Is Possible

When a person has a chronic condition like multiple sclerosis, daily long-term skilled help with health and personal needs may be in order. Whatever level of care is needed, it can take place in three settings:

- the person's own home
- your home
- residential care facilities, such as a foster care home, assisted living, or a skilled nursing facility

Home Care Considerations

Whether care will take place in your home or in the home of the person who needs care, the following factors must be considered:

- Is there enough room for both the person and items such as a wheelchair, walker, bedside toilet, and lift?

- How accessible is the home if walkers or wheelchairs are used?

- Is a doctor, nurse, or specialist available to supervise care when needed?

- Is there a hospital emergency unit close by?

- Is the home environment safe and supportive and does it allow for some independence?

- Is money available to hire additional help?

- Is the person in question willing to have a caregiver in the home?

- Can the caregiver manage this role along with other family and personal responsibilities?

Things That Must Be Provided

- medication

- meals

- personal care

- housecleaning

- shopping

- transportation

- companionship

- accessibility (wheelchair ramps, support railings, and changes to the bath and shower stall) (📖 See *Preparing the Home,* p. 109)

Benefits of Home Care

- When a caregiver's spouse is supportive, the experience can strengthen the marriage.

- The relationship between the caregiver and the person in care can grow stronger.

- A great deal of money can be saved on health care costs.

Why Home Care May Not Be Possible

- financial reasons (inadequate health insurance to cover the cost of home nursing)
- family limits (lack of time or money)
- the caregiver's lack of physical and emotional strength
- the person's complex medical condition
- the home's physical layout
- the person's desire to live independently of family

Possible Hazards of Home Care

- Possible lack of freedom for the caregiver.
- Caregiver duties may affect the caregiver's job, career, hobbies, and personal life.
- There may be less time for family members, and the caregiver's family relationships may suffer.
- Children in the home may need to be quieter.
- There may be less time for religious services and volunteer work.
- Friends and family may criticize the caregiver's efforts and offer unwelcome advice.
- The caregiver may often be awakened during the night.
- The caregiver may feel unable to control life's events and may suffer from depression, worry, anger, regrets, guilt, and stress.
- Instead of being grateful, the person receiving care may display unpleasant changes in attitude.
- He or she may react to constant daily irritations by lashing out at the caregiver.

- The caregiver may begin to fear the time when he or she may be dependent on someone for care.

- The caregiver may feel obliged to spend personal funds on caregiving.

- The caregiver may become physically ill and emotionally drained.

Outside Help

One of the biggest pitfalls in caregiving is trying to do it all yourself. But other help is available and should be called on whenever possible. That help includes:

- support groups

- day care and respite care, which provide relief for the caregiver

- organizations providing respite care

- pastoral counseling services

- parish nurses

- medical services provided by professionals, such as nurses and therapists

- personal services for the person in your care, such as grooming or dressing, provided by home health aides

- community home health services on a fee basis, such as Visiting Nurse Associations (📖 See *Getting In-Home Help,* p. 78)

Supportive Housing and Care Options

If you believe that home care is not practical for you, many other options exist. Good programs foster independence, dignity, privacy, a very high level of functioning, and connections with the community. However, people who have lived independently all their lives may not be

Checklist **The Ideal Caregiver**

The ideal caregiver is—

✓ *emotionally and physically capable of handling the work*

✓ *able to share duties and responsibilities with other willing family members*

✓ *able to plan solutions and solve problems instead of withdrawing under stress*

✓ *able to speak in a simple and clear way*

✓ *comfortable giving and receiving help*

✓ *trained for the level of care required*

✓ *able to handle unpleasant tasks such as changing diapers, bathing, or cleaning bed sores*

✓ *in good health and has energy, skill, and the ability to adapt*

✓ *able to cope with anger and frustration*

✓ *able to afford respite (back-up) care when necessary*

✓ *able to speak to and understand the care receiver*

✓ *able to make this person feel useful and needed*

✓ *valued by other family members*

✓ *able to adjust to the future needs and wishes of the person in care*

✓ *aware of other care options and willing to explore them*

If you have most of these traits, you may be a good candidate to provide home care.

suited to live in groups, and those who are mentally alert or are younger may be very unhappy living with people who suffer from dementia.

Keep the above factors in mind when you check out the following:

- **Independent Living Options**—apartment buildings, condos, retirement communities, and single-family homes

- **Semi-independent Living Options**—places that offer the same benefits as independent living but also include meal service and housekeeping as part of the monthly fee, provide help with personal care, keep track of health and medications, and provide special diets. These options are frequently offered in assisted living facilities and group homes.

- **Skilled Care Facilities**—nursing homes

 States use different names for care facilities. The services can also vary, so it is important to check with the facility and each state's licensing agency to confirm exactly which services are offered. For example, in Wyoming, assisted living allows people who are unrelated to share a room. In some other places, living spaces are not shared, except by personal choice.

A Closer Look at the Options

House Sharing—for people who are fully independent

- Two or more unrelated people live together, each with a private bedroom.

- All living areas are shared.

- Chores and expenses are shared.

- Personal-assistant services may be shared.

Group Homes or Adult Foster Care Homes—homes in residential neighborhoods for people whose needs vary, from assistance with individual services to dependent residents with increased nursing services

- Care is given to small groups of people in the primary caregiver's home or with a live-in resident manager/caregiver.

- The home is privately run and provides private or shared rooms with meals, housekeeping, personal care (such as bathing and dressing), keeping track of medication, safety supervision, and some transportation.

- Rates vary according to individual care needs, and Medicaid funding is often available for repayment to those who qualify.

- Staff are qualified and facilities are licensed according to the level of services offered, which can include housekeeping, laundry, personal care assistance, bathing, dressing, grooming, and management of medication and other medical needs, such as injections or inability to control bladder and bowel.

NOTE Some states do not license, inspect, or keep watch over adult foster care homes. Before selecting one, call your local Area Agency on Aging or the state or county Department of Health to see if any complaints have been filed against the home you are considering.

Assisted Living Facilities—for moderate assistance to those who are frail and usually require assistance with activities of daily living

- Each person lives in his or her own apartment.

- An emergency staff is available 24 hours a day.

- Monthly charges are based on the level of service needed.

- Activities such as games, hobbies, crafts, and music are offered.

- Meals, housekeeping, medication management, and nursing assessment are provided.

- Transportation and access to medical services can be arranged.

> **NOTE** There is no national control over these facilities but there is state licensing and regulation. For information on a specific facility, call the ombudsman in your state or the state agency that licenses the facility. (An ombudsman is someone who looks into complaints made by individuals.)

Continuing Care Retirement Communities—for people who want a range of services from independent living to nursing home care

- These facilities provide a lifetime contract for care.

- They provide or offer meals and can handle special diets.

- They offer housekeeping, scheduled transportation, emergency help, personal care, and activities for fun and learning.

- Many retirement communities require entrance fees that can vary quite a bit.

- They also have monthly fees ranging from several hundred to several thousand dollars.

- Some provide home health care and nursing home care without extra fees.

- Some charge extra for nursing unit residents.

Nursing Homes—for people who require continuous and ongoing nursing assistance or monitoring

Nursing homes typically offer three levels of care:

- **Custodial**—minimal nursing, but help with hygiene, meals, dressing, etc.

- **Intermediate**—help for those who cannot live alone but do not need 24-hour skilled nursing care

- **Skilled Nursing**—intensive 24-hour skilled nursing care

Hospice care is available in all settings as a covered benefit under Medicare. It is also covered for those who receive Medicaid in states that offer hospice coverage under their Medicaid program.

Financing Options

The choice of the right housing option may depend on financing available:

- **Personal Resources** are the most common way to pay.

- **Private Insurance** is helpful, but some policies limit the length and type of benefits and have waiting periods or other limits.

- **Medicare** is for those 65 and older or for people who have been declared disabled by the Social Security Administration. Medicare partially pays for up to 100 days in a skilled nursing care facility after a qualifying related hospitalization of more than three days in a row (not including the day the person leaves the hospital). The financing of hospice care is a separate benefit under Medicare.

- **Medicaid** partially pays for services, including assisted living services in some states, to those who are aged, blind, or have disabilities and have limited financial resources. It is also a major payer for nursing home care.

Checklist **Review Before Deciding on a Facility**

✓ Is a trial period allowed to be sure a person is happy with the facility?

✓ Will the facility refund deposits or entrance fees if the resident dies, chooses to leave, or is asked to leave?

✓ Can a resident choose his or her own apartment? Can personal furniture be used?

✓ Are there younger residents at the facility?

✓ If the person must be away for a short time (even for a hospital stay), will the same apartment be available when he or she returns? Is there a reduced rate during long absences?

✓ If the person marries, can the couple live in the same apartment?

✓ Can the staff handle special diets? Are meal menus posted?

✓ Is transportation provided?

✓ How many people are on staff and how much training have they had?

✓ How often and for what reasons can staff enter the apartment?

✓ Can the resident see his or her own doctor? Who gives out the medications?

✓ Is physical therapy available within the facility?

✓ Is the facility licensed to deal with a resident whose health gets worse or must the person leave if, for example, he or she can no longer walk or begins arguing or fighting with others?

✓ How are decisions made when a person must be moved to another part of the facility?

✓ Is there a 30-day-notice provision for ending the agreement?

✓ Does the facility take Medicare?

✓ Will the facility let a resident "spend down" his or her assets and go on Medicaid?

- **Medigap** policies cover gaps in coverage and may be in place to pay Medicare coinsurance.

Points to Review Before Signing a Contract or Lease

Although it is hard to know what problems may arise in a care setting, it is extremely important to take the following steps before signing any legal papers:

- Find out who owns the facility and review the owner's financial status.

- Ask for a copy of the contract and review it with an attorney or financial advisor.

- Do not rely on spoken promises. Make sure the contract is geared to the resident's needs.

- Read the state inspection report on the facility.

- Read all the rules and policies of the facility that are not in the contract.

- Ask to see the facility's license.

Things You Should Know About Facilities

Residents' Rights

General Rights—Residents maintain all their rights guaranteed under the U.S. Constitution, including the right to vote. In addition, they can receive visitors, voice their concerns, form resident councils, and enjoy informed consent, privacy, and freedom of choice.

Privacy—In some cases, a resident may have a roommate. However, residents' rooms are considered private and staff must knock before entering. Also, residents can have private visits with spouses.

Restraints—Only the resident's doctor may order a restraint as part of a care plan and must state the specific restraint's use and period of use. (Use of restraints is strongly discouraged, although not prohibited.)

Lifestyle Choices—Residents do not have as many choices as they would have at home regarding meal times, menu choices, and times for sleep. However, most facilities try to satisfy residents' needs as much as possible.

Ability to Effect Change—Issues can be brought up to the resident council or the long-term-care ombudsman.

Freedom to Leave—A person chooses to enter a facility and has the right to leave at any time regardless of what the family thinks or safety concerns.

 The following describes general guidelines regarding a resident's rights. To obtain specific rules for a particular state, contact the state agency responsible for licensing the facility.

The Resident's Rights When Leaving a Facility

Depending on the admission agreement, a resident must be given written notice 30 days before being moved. If there is a medical emergency, no written notice is required. Generally, a resident may be moved from a facility for the following reasons:

- The person wants to be moved.
- The person must be moved for his or her own good.
- The person must be moved for the good of other residents.
- The facility is not being paid. (However, someone who runs out of money cannot be moved *if* Medicaid will pay.)

- The person came into the facility for special care and that care is completed.

- The facility is being closed.

If the person does not want to leave the facility, IMMEDI-ATELY contact the state agency responsible for licensing the facility and/or Medicaid certification.

If you have questions, call the following:

- the Center for Medicare-Medicaid Services

- the local Senior and Disabled Services Division of the Department of Health and Human Resources

- the long-term-care ombudsman

- the Federal Health Care Financing Administration

- the local Area Agency on Aging

What Family Members and Friends Should Do

- Visit whenever possible.

- Send cards or letters between visits.

- Bring small gifts and treats.

- If allowed, walk around with the person when visiting to provide exercise.

- Listen to the resident's complaints.

- Build a good relationship with the staff.

- Plan off-site outings if appropriate.

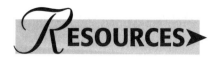

RESOURCES

AARP
601 E Street, NW
Washington, DC 20049
(800) 424-3410
www.aarp.org
*Web site provides information on housing and other
senior issues.*

National Council on Independent Living
1916 Wilson Boulevard, Suite 209
Arlington, VA 22201
(703) 525-3406 (voice)
(703) 525-4153 (tty)
ncil@ncil.org
www.ncil.org
*Refers callers to local independent-living centers. Offers
publications and advice related to disability issues. Advo-
cates for policy changes.*

Assisted Living Facilities and Nursing Homes

**American Association of Homes and Services
for the Aging**
2519 Connecticut Avenue, NW
Washington, DC 20008
(202) 783-2255
(800) 508-9442
www.aahsa.org
*Provides information on not-for-profit nursing homes, se-
nior housing facilities, assisted living, and community services. Call for free consumer information brochure.*

American Health Care Association/National Center for Assisted Living
1201 L Street, NW
Washington, DC 20005
(202) 842-4444
www.ahca.org
Provides consumer information on services, financing, public policy, nursing facilities, assisted living, and subacute care. Represents more than 10,000 providers of assisted living, nursing care, and subacute care.

Assisted Living Federation of America
11200 Waples Mill Road, Suite 150
Fairfax, VA 22030
(703) 691-8100
www.alfa.org
Offers referrals to local facilities listed by state. Provides free 15-page consumer guide to assisted living.

The Center for Medicare and Medicaid Services has detailed information about the past performance of every Medicare- and Medicaid-certified nursing home in the country. For more information, go to www.medicare.gov, click on Search Tools at the top of the page, and then click on Compare Nursing Homes in Your Area. For a list of **Medicare-certified nursing homes**, call the local office of the Department on Aging.

Respite Services

ARCH National Respite Locator Service
800 Eastowne Drive, Suite 105
Chapel Hill, NC 27514-2204
(919) 490-5577
www.respitelocator.org
Provides caregivers with contact information on respite services in their area.

55

Eldercare Locator
National Association of Area Agencies on Aging
1730 Rhode Island Avenue, NW, Suite 1200
Washington, DC 20036
(800) 677-1116
www.eldercare.gov
www.aoa.dhhs.gov
Supplies information about many eldercare issues, including respite care. Provides referrals to local respite programs and local Area Agency on Aging.

If you don't have access to the Internet, ask your local library to help you locate a Web site.

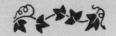

Using the Health Care Team Effectively

Using the Health Care Team Effectively

*W*hen you care for someone in the home, you must also manage that person's health care. This means choosing a good medical team, keeping costs down, arranging for medical appointments, and getting the best, least expensive medicines. It also means knowing what the insurance rules are and, most important, being an advocate (a supporter) for the person in your care.

Doctors and nurses can focus on physical diagnosis and may ignore the emotional aspects of care. Sometimes they have little time to consider the spiritual aspects of healing. Although you should consult with professionals about the levels of therapy and support needed for the person in your care, you do not have to accept what they suggest or order. Keep asking questions until you completely understand the diagnosis (what is wrong), treatment, and prognosis (likely outcome).

Who Makes Up the Stroke Health Care Team?

Very few survivors get better all by themselves. Surviving and then recovering from a stroke require many different people involved in a long chain of survival and recovery. There is no guarantee that a stroke survivor will get better as a result of the care provided by these professionals, but it can be safely said that very few survivors get better all by themselves.

There are four stages of care: acute, acute rehab, subacute rehab, and at-home rehab. Each stage will be explained in the text that follows.

Moving from one care team to another is often not well coordinated and this is where you, as caregiver, can be very helpful. Your survivor will do much better in the healthcare system when you communicate information from one team to another. There is a trend toward electronic record keeping, but it is not currently the norm and may not be for a decade. Generally what travels between facilities is a written chart, which is often illegible. Consider it part of your job as caregiver to give important information to those responsible at each facility. Although each facility will do its own assessment, it is important for you to communicate all that you know about your survivor's condition to each person in the new healthcare team.

 For starters, make a hand-written or typed list of your survivor's deficits (physical, cognitive, speech) and medications, and provide it to each new facility or unit he or she is moved to. Save this list, if possible in your computer, and update it when necessary so that it's always current. Be sure to take the medication list or chart to every doctor's appointment.

Acute Stage

The professionals at work during this stage of care may well save your survivor's life. As the caregiver, you won't have much interaction with this group. Think of your survivor's care as a chain of survival, and each professional is a link in that chain.

- **EMT**—The emergency technicians who respond to your medical emergency and will work to stabilize the person having the stroke.

- **ER Nurse**—The emergency room nurse monitors the patient, administers medications, and ensures procedures are carried out as ordered by the ER physician; the ER nurse also documents the patient's care.

- **ER Physician**—This doctor performs the first physical exam, works to stabilize the patient, and orders any tests or scans needed for diagnosis.

- **Neurologist**—This brain doctor takes over once a stroke diagnosis is given.

- **Neuroradiologist**—This specialist uses radioactive substances, X rays, and scanning devices to diagnose diseases of the nervous system.

- **Interventional radiologist**—This physician uses scanning technology to guide the delivery and use of balloons, as well as catheters with drugs and stents for treatment of acute stroke.

- **Neurosurgeon**—Treatment for some strokes, particularly broken-artery (hemorrhagic) strokes, involves brain surgery.

NOTE **Dial 9-1-1 if you observe stroke symptoms**. Tell the dispatcher that the person is having a stroke.

Don't take the person to the hospital yourself. Here's why—

1. He will probably get there sooner by ambulance.

2. The emergency personnel will begin to stabilize the patient immediately.

3. A recent study showed that stroke patients who arrive at the hospital by ambulance receive more appropriate care more quickly. Have the person's chart and list of medications ready when the ambulance comes; and don't forget if there is an Advance Directive (a legal document stating a person's healthcare preferences.)

Acute Rehab Stage

To be admitted to acute rehabilitation, your survivor must be able to do three hours of rehab a day—90 minutes of physical therapy and 90 minutes of occupational therapy. The links in this part of the chain include:

- **Physiatrist** (fe-zi-a-trist)—A physician specializing in physical medicine and rehabilitation. He or she is responsible for assessing a patient's rehab needs, designing a rehab program, and deciding how long the patient stays in rehab. The physiatrist becomes the primary doctor during this stage of recovery.

- **Rehabilitation psychologist**—A psychologist who works with people with disabilities to assess the psychological aspects of the disability and help survivors reach the highest level of physical, mental, and personal function possible.

- **Physical therapist**—A PT works with survivors' large muscles to improve strength, balance, and function.

- **Occupational therapist**—An OT works with survivors' fine-motor control to improve quality of life.

- **Speech therapist**—Speech therapy involves all aspects of communication. In addition to speech, this therapist may work with reading, writing, and other cognitive functions, as well as swallowing.

> **NOTE** Rehab makes a difference in your survivor's and your quality of life. *In order for insurance to continue to pay for rehab, survivors must show progress.* Once the survivor plateaus, insurance stops paying. The deciding factor is not whether you or your survivor feel rehab is helping, but whether she is making *measurable progress*. For this reason, encourage your survivor and *document her progress*. Advocate for your survivor with the therapists and make sure *every* improvement is noted in her records. Failure to make progress in rehab may be a sign of depression. Rehab should be put on hold until the depression is treated.

Sub-acute Rehab Stage

Sub-acute rehab is for survivors who can't go home and who can't perform three hours of rehab daily. Usually, people in these skilled nursing facilities receive an hour to 90 minutes of rehab a day. Although orders for care will come from a doctor, the family or caregiver will generally interact with nurses and therapists. The links in this part of the chain are allied healthcare professionals (medical professionals who work together to achieve a common goal) such as PTs, OTs, speech therapists, and nurses.

At-Home Care Stage

There are many levels of outpatient care programs. In some, therapists come to the home to deliver therapy, others may require the survivor to go into a facility. Either way, it will be a therapist and not a doctor who is involved with the survivor and family caregiver on a day-to-day basis. At this stage of recovery, your survivor may only see a physiatrist every two or three months to evaluate progress and (it is hoped) write another prescription for therapy.

 For almost a decade, Congress has tried to impose strict caps on Medicare coverage for outpatient physical, occupational, and speech therapy. When first introduced in 1997, the cap was $1,500 each for physical and speech therapy. However, public outrage prompted Congress to pass a moratorium on implementation of the caps, not once but twice. The second moratorium expired in December 2005, and Medicare immediately imposed a $1,740 cap on outpatient physical therapy and speech-language pathology benefits *combined*. Fortunately, therapy for stroke was given an automatic exemption.

How to Share in Medical Decisions

In the end, medical decision-making is in the hands of the stroke survivor, the doctor, and the caregiver. Learn to take an active role and become an advocate for yourself and for the person in your care. It has been said that a patient is the senior partner in the patient–doctor relationship.

Long-Range Considerations

- Find out how the person in your care feels about treatments that prolong life. Respect these views.

- Help the person receiving care to set up an advance directive and power of attorney for health care.

- Share decisions with the doctor and the care receiver and take responsibility for the treatment and its outcomes.

The Doctor–Patient–Caregiver Relationship

- Be aware that doctors must see more patients per day than they once did.

- Be aware that some doctors may have financial reasons for doing too much or too little for those in their care. Specialists are often the only ones with the training needed to treat a serious or chronic condition, so the doctor may refer the survivor to a specialist.

- If the relationship with the doctor becomes unfriendly, find a new doctor.

- Respect the doctor's time (you may need to have more than one visit to cover all issues).

- If Medicare is the payer, ask if the doctor accepts Medicare assignment. If not, the difference may have to be paid out of pocket.

Preparing for a Visit to the Doctor

- Be prepared to briefly explain the care receiver's and the family's medical history.

- Take a list of questions in order of importance.

- Prepare a list of any symptoms the person you care for is experiencing.

- Be prepared to ask for written information on the medical situation so you can better understand what the doctor is saying, or bring a small tape recorder.

- You can call the hospital's library or health resource center for help in looking up any questions the doctor does not answer.

Be sure shots for tetanus, flu, and pneumonia are up-to-date. For those on Medicare, flu and pneumonia shots are covered.

At the Doctor's Office

- Tell the doctor what you hope and expect from the visit and any recommended treatment.

- If the doctor tells you to do something you know you can't do, such as give medication in the middle of the night, ask if there is another treatment and explain why.

- Insist on talking about the level of care that you believe is appropriate and that agrees with the care receiver's wishes.

- Ask about other options for tests, medications, and surgery.

- Ask why tests or treatments are needed and what the risks are.

- Consider all options, including the pros and cons of "watchful waiting."

- Trust your common sense and if you have doubts, get a second opinion.

Questions to Ask Before Agreeing to Tests and Medications

Before you begin discussing medical treatment with the doctor, explain that the person in your care does not want any unnecessary tests or treatments. Then ask these questions:

- Why is this test needed?

- How long will it take? How soon will the results be in?

- Is the test accurate?

- Is it painful?

- Are there risks with the treatment? Do the benefits outweigh the risks?

- How long will side effects occur and how long will they last?

- Are X rays really needed?

- Will the doctor review the test report and explain it in detail?

- May a copy of the report be taken home? (If you have questions, ask to talk to the specialist who made the report.)

- If a test is positive, what course of action should be taken?

- Is the condition going to worsen slowly or rapidly?

- What could happen if the person did not have the test?

- How much does the test cost and is there a less costly one?

Questions to Ask the Doctor About Medications

Medications can be costly, confusing to use, and have unwanted side effects. Be sure to ask questions when medicines are prescribed and prescriptions are filled.

- Give the doctor a list of all medications and dosages that the person in your care is now taking, including eye drops, vitamins, and herbal remedies.

- Tell the doctor of any other treatments being used. Sometimes using two or more treatments may be fatal or may keep the new treatment from working.

- Tell the doctor of any allergies or if there are certain foods the person cannot eat (food allergies).

- Understand why each medication is needed and how much it will help the person's condition.

- Ask if pain can be relieved almost completely, and then ask for the medicine that works best.

- Ask how long it takes for the drug to work.

- Find out its side effects.

- Ask if the drug could react with other drugs and what you should do if there are side effects.

- Find out if a change in diet, exercise, reducing stress, or other things can be done.

- If more than one medicine is needed, ask the doctor if they can be taken at the same times each day. If a drug must be taken at a difficult time (for instance, in the middle of the night), ask about another choice.

- Try to find the lowest cost drug. Ask if a generic (non-brand name) drug or another brand in the same drug class is available at a lower cost.

- Be sure that the generic drug will not have a poor effect on the person's condition.

- Ask if a lower dose can be prescribed without bad effects.

- To keep costs down, ask if a higher dose can be safely prescribed and the pill cut in half.

- Ask if you can buy a one-week supply of a new medication to see if the person can handle any possible side effects. Or ask if the physician has free samples to try.

Tip

BUYING MEDICATIONS

Buying medications through mail order is often the cheapest way to buy. Ask if the insurance company has a mail-order program (*see Resources,* p. 76).

Questions to Ask the Pharmacist

Some prescription drugs are not covered by health insurance, so shop around for the drug store with the lowest prices, and then stay with it. The pharmacist will come to know the care receiver's condition and can advise you about problems that might come up. Managed care plans are permitted to change doctor's orders by giving you a similar version that is cheaper. Do not try cutting drug costs without talking to you doctor about it first.

- Find out the highest allowable charge for a particular drug.

- Ask what over-the-counter drugs the pharmacist suggests for the person's condition (it may be necessary to take more of the drug if it is over-the-counter).

- Ask if the insurance company will pay for the drug the doctor prescribed.

- Ask if the doctor will be called to approve the switch to another drug.

- Find out what generic drug can be used instead of the prescription drug.

- Ask if the generic drug can cause side effects and when the doctor should be called about them.

- Ask if using more than one drug can cause unsafe drug interactions.

- Ask if the pharmacy's computer will alert the pharmacist about drug-interactions or side effects before the prescription is filled.

- Find out the risks of not taking the medicine.

- Find out the risks of not finishing the prescription.

- If you are caring for someone who will be taking several medications on his or her own, find a drug store that has easy-to-use packaging.

- Ask if the medicine can be put in a large easy-to-open container with a label in large print.

- Ask if an overdose of the medicine is dangerous.

- Ask if the person can drink alcohol or smoke while taking the medication.

- Ask if the medicine must be taken with a meal, with water or milk, etc.

- When the person needs many expensive drugs, find out if you can get a discount or work out a payment plan.

MEDICAL ALERT
A survivor may want to wear a medical alert bracelet, or carry a card, that lists the medications he or she is currently taking.

MEDICAL RECORDS
To save costs, have all medical records and tests sent to the second doctor. Also, if possible, bring the important ones with you.

 Even the experts can disagree about the best treatment. The final decision is yours.

Mental Health Treatment

Strong emotions are a normal part of long-term illness. Counseling and support groups are a very helpful way of dealing with these feelings.

- For one who is depressed and needs therapy, ask the primary care doctor to give you the name of a therapist.

- Be aware that many people are embarrassed about mental health problems and may not want to seek care.

Dental Care

Dental care is important for overall wellness. For low-cost dental programs, check with university dental schools or the local Area Agency on Aging.

- Tell the dentist all the medications the person is taking before starting dental treatment.

- Try to go to a dentist who is familiar with the person's disease.

- Find out how many visits will be needed each year.

- Ask if the office and dental chair are accessible, if that is needed.

- Ask about low-cost options to the treatment the dentist suggests.

- Ask if X rays are really necessary.

- Find out the cost of dentures, but don't trust prices that seem too good to be true. Cheap dentures may not fit correctly.

- When seeking another opinion, have all medical records and tests sent to the second dentist.

Vision Care

Regular eye exams every two years by a specialist in eye disease (ophthalmologist) or someone who examines the eyes (optometrist) are necessary. These exams can also spot or detect other serious diseases such as diabetes. Finding and treating disease early can prevent serious diseases from getting worse and leading to blindness.

- Tell the doctor of any medicines the person is taking.

- Tell the doctor if there is a family history of glaucoma.

- Get a yearly eye exam for a person with diabetes.

- Contact your state's Commission for the Blind for information on self-help organizations for those with low vision.

- Ask for help in finding products ("talking" watches, etc.) and aids that will help the person adjust to low vision.

- Seek out radio stations that have programs of newspaper readings.

NOTE Danger signs to watch for are changes in the color or size of an object when one eye is covered or when straight poles appear bent or wavy. See an ophthalmologist (eye doctor) without delay.

How to Watch Out for Someone's Best Interests in the Hospital

A person in the hospital is at greater risk than others, so be ready to keep tabs on treatments, ask questions, and act as an advocate.

- If the Patients' Bill of Rights is not posted in a place where it can be seen, ask for a copy.

- Agree only to treatments that have been thoroughly explained.

- If something is not being done and you think it should be, ask why.

- Be friendly and show respect to hospital staff. They will probably respond better to you and to the person in your care. Bad feelings between family members and staff may cause the staff to avoid the person.

- Assist with the person's grooming and care.

- Speak up if you notice doctors or nurses examining anyone without first washing their hands.

- Check all bills and ask questions about anything that isn't clear to you.

> **NOTE** According to federal law, a hospital must release patients in a *safe manner* or else must keep them in the hospital. Letting a patient leave the hospital is not wise if the person has constant fever, infection, or pain that cannot be controlled, confusion, disorientation (no sense of time or place), or is unable to take food and liquids by mouth. However, in some cases, it may be better for the person to be released because the noise and risk of catching other diseases may make it more difficult to recover. If you plan to appeal a discharge, understand the rules of Medicare, Medicaid, the HMO, or insurance plan.

When You Doubt the Time Is Right for Discharge

- State your doubts in a simple letter to the hospital's director or the health plan's medical director. (Rules vary from state to state.)

- Meet with the hospital's discharge planner.

- Ask if the hospital is following the usual policy for the condition.

- Explain any special reasons that make you think it is unwise to discharge the person.

Checklist **Coming Home from the Hospital**

✓ Assess the person's condition and needs.

✓ Understand the diagnosis (what is wrong) and prognosis (what will happen).

✓ Become part of the health care team (doctor, nurse, therapists) so you can learn how to provide care.

✓ Get complete written instructions from the doctor. If there is anything you don't understand, ASK QUESTIONS.

✓ Arrange follow-up care from the doctor.

✓ Develop a plan of care with the doctor. (📖 See **Setting Up a Plan of Care**, p. 153.)

✓ Meet with the hospital's social worker or discharge planner to determine home care benefits.

✓ Understand in-home assistance options. (📖 See **Getting In-Home Help**, p. 78.)

✓ Arrange for in-home help.

✓ Arrange physical, occupational, and speech therapy as needed.

✓ Find out if medicine is provided by the hospital to take home. If not, you will have to have prescriptions filled before you take the person home.

✓ Prepare the home. (📖 See **Preparing the Home**, p. 109.)

✓ Buy needed supplies; rent, borrow, or buy equipment such as wheelchairs, crutches, and walkers.

✓ Take home all personal items.

✓ Check with the hospital cashier for discharge payment requirements.

✓ Arrange transportation (an ambulance or van if your car will not do).

- Ask if the hospital rules can be changed to cover this special case.

- Remember that anyone has the right to appeal a discharge.

- Get your doctor's help in the appeal, but understand that he or she may have different reasons for wanting to discharge the person.

 Do not hesitate to call the hospital staff member (ombudsman) who is responsible for patients' rights.

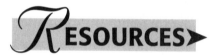

For free or low-cost resources, contact local consumer health resource and information centers (check the local hospital system or phone book) and local health agencies or associations (American Heart Association, American Diabetes Association, and others).

Doctor's Guide to the Internet—Patient Edition
www.pslgroup.com/PTGUIDE.HTM
Provides information for specific diseases and gives pointers to other Internet sites of medical information.

Go Ask Alice!
www.goaskalice.columbia.edu/about.html
Provides helpful information and lets you post health-related questions.

The Health Resource, Inc.
933 Faulkner Street
Conway, AR 72034
(800) 949-0090; (501) 329-5272; Fax (501) 329-9489
www.thehealthresource.com
Provides clients with personalized detailed reports on their specific medical conditions. These reports contain conventional and alternative treatments and information on current research, nutrition, self-help measures, specialists, and resource organizations. Reports on any non-cancer condition are $295, or $395 for complex issues, and contain 50 to 100 pages. Reports on any cancer condition are $395 and contain 150 to 200 pages. Shipping is additional.

University of Washington
www.uwmedicine.org
A great storehouse of general health information on all topics.

Information About Eyesight

Lighthouse International
111 E. 59th Street
New York, NY 10022
(800) 829-0500
www.lighthouse.org

Lions Club International
300 W. 22nd Street
Oak Brook, IL 60523
www.lionsclub.org
(630) 571-5466

National Association for Visually Handicapped
22 West 21st Street, 6th floor
New York, NY 10010
(212) 889-3141
www.navh.org

National Federation of the Blind
1800 Johnson Street
Baltimore, MD 21230
(410) 659-9314
www.nfb.org

Publication

A *Family Caregiver's Guide to Hospital Discharge Planning,* a publication of the National Alliance for Caregiving and the United Hospital Fund of New York. Available at www.caregiving.org

If you don't have access to the Internet, ask your local library to help you locate a Web site.

Medications

Together Rx Access™ Card
A joint program by drug companies offering a free Prescription Savings Card for individuals and families who meet all four of the following requirements:

❏ Not eligible for Medicare
❏ Have no public or private prescription-drug coverage
❏ Household income equal to or less than:
—$30,000 for a single person
—$40,000 for a family of two
—$50,000 for a family of three
—$60,000 for a family of four
—$70,000 for a family of five

❏ Legal resident of the U.S. or Puerto Rico

Call 1-800-250-2839 to begin saving on your prescriptions. For the most current list of medicines and products, visit www.TogetherRxAccess.com

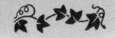

Getting In-Home Help

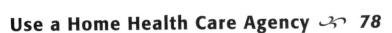

Getting In-Home Help

$\mathcal{G}$etting help with caregiving in the home involves the following options:

- *Using a home health care agency (typical fee range: $50 to $150 per visit through a private agency)*

- *Hiring someone privately (typical fee range: $12 to $15 per hour; the cost of assistance is based on the category of professional or his or her experience)*

- *Performing all caregiving duties with the assistance of family and friends.*

Use a Home Health Care Agency

Home Health Care Agencies are for-profit, nonprofit, or are run by the government. They provide personal care, skilled care, instructions for caregiver and care receiver, and supervision. They usually provide certified nurse assistants (CNAs), sometimes called home health aides; registered nurses (RNs); licensed practical nurses (LPNs); physical therapists, occupational therapists, and speech therapists. (A doctor's order is required in order to get coverage for skilled-care nursing in the home.) These agencies help plan services and care that match the health, social, and financial needs of the client.

Definitions for Agencies

There are a number of terms to describe an agency's services and how it is able to do what it does. Study the terms carefully before looking into the agencies in your area.

Accredited—Services have been reviewed by a nonprofit organization interested in quality home health care.

Bonded—The agency has paid a fixed dollar amount in order to be bonded. In the event of a court action the bond pays the penalties. (Being bonded does not ensure good service.)

Certified—The agency has met the lowest federal standards for care and takes part in the Medicare program.

Certified Health Personnel—Those who work for the agency meet the standards of a licensing agency for the state.

Insurance Claims Honored—The agency will look into insurance benefits and will accept assignment of benefits (meaning the insurance company pays the agency directly).

Licensed—The agency has met the requirements to run its business (in those states that oversee home health care agencies).

Licensed Health Personnel—The personnel (staff) of the agency have passed the state licensing exam for that profession.

Screened—References have been checked; a criminal background check may or may not have been made.

How to Pay for Using an Agency

Paying for care from an agency ranges from Medicare to private pay to long-term-care insurance to state and county programs.

Medicare

To be eligible for the Medicare home-health benefit, a person must be basically unable to leave the house (homebound) and need skilled care.

- Medicare pays the full cost of medically necessary home health visits by a Medicare-approved home health agency.

- Medicare and most insurers will pay for skilled care (such as a registered nurse) that is not for maintenance.

- The person must be as unable to care for himself or herself as someone who would be in a nursing home.

 NOTE State rules vary on who is eligible, so check with your area Medicare office for local rules.

State and County Personal Assistance Programs

- The person receiving services may need to be certified as eligible for a nursing home.

- Many programs require that the person be at a low-income level.

- Funding may come from Medicaid waivers and funding is sometimes not regular.

Private Pay

- If a person does not qualify for public funds, he or she must pay with long-term-care insurance or pay privately.

- Care management through Area Agencies on Aging may be free or offered on a sliding scale, based on a person's income.

What the Home Health Care Agency Will Do

- carry out an in-home visit

- look into insurance benefits and publicly funded benefits

- ask for an assignment of benefits (where payments are made by the insurer directly to the agency)

- ask you to sign a form to release medical information

- ask you to agree to and sign a service contract

- carry out an assessment (by the director of nurses) to determine the level of care required

- discuss the costs of suggested services

- come up with a plan of care that shows the person's diagnosis (what is wrong), functional limitations (what the person can and cannot do), medications, special diet, what services are provided by agency, advice for care, and list of equipment needed

- give you a written copy of the plan of care

- send a copy of the plan of care to the person's doctor

- select and send the right caregivers, only to the level of care needed, to the person's home

- adjust services to meet changing needs

Expect the Agency to:

- be an advocate, advisor, and service planner and to share information clearly with you

- give a full professional assessment

- get in touch with the care receiver's doctor as part of the assessment process

- have knowledge of long-term-care services and how to pay for them

- fill out the paperwork for publicly funded benefits

- show no bias or favor to service providers who may have contracts with the agency

- provide confidential treatment that will not be talked about with others

Checklist **Things to Do Before Selecting an Agency**

✔ Interview several agencies.

✔ Get references and CHECK THEM.

✔ Make a list of services you want and ask the agency what it will cost.

✔ Ask what the steps are in the care planning and management process and how long each will take.

✔ Find out how and when you can contact the care manager.

✔ Find out if the agency has a system for sending a substitute (stand-in) aide if the regular one doesn't show up.

✔ Ask if the agency will replace the aide if that aide and the person in care do not get along.

✔ Ask about the skills and ongoing training of personnel.

✔ Ask how they keep track of the quality of services.

✔ Ask for the services needed by the person in care, even if the insurance company is trying to hold down costs.

✔ Be aware that if a social service agency is providing the care services, they may limit you to only the services that they provide.

✔ Ask them to tell you about any referral-fee agreements they may have with nursing homes or other care facilities.

✔ Know what you have to do to lodge complaints against the agency with the state ombudsman or long-term-care office.

✔ Get in touch with the local/state Division for Aging Services to check for complaints against a particular agency.

- provide a written account of care when you ask for it

- have a proven track record of being honest, reliable, and trusted if the agency handles a person's money

Hire Someone Privately—A Personal Assistant

Even if you decide not to use an agency, a health care professional can help you decide how to prepare the home. They can give advice about needed supplies and where to purchase them and set up a care program. However, when you hire someone privately, you must assume payroll responsibility, complete required government forms (such as Social Security), decide on fringe benefits, track travel expenses, and provide a detailed list of tasks to be done.

Tip

WHEN YOU START CALLING FOR RESOURCES:

- Have information ready, such as what services will be needed and personal information, such as the age of the person, date of birth, social security number, etc.).

- Have your questions written down and ready.

- Realize that to be eligible for some services there may be income, age, or geographic requirements.

- COMMUNICATE, COMMUNICATE, COMMUNICATE what you want and need!

Where to Find Help

- Yellow Pages under Nurses, Nursing Services, Social Service Organizations, Home Health Services, and Senior Services

- commercial agencies, which operate like temp employment agencies, screen applicants, and provide you with a list of candidates

- nonprofit agencies, such as the Visiting Nurse Association, which may charge a fee on a sliding scale (based on ability to pay)
- public health nursing through a county social service department (if you have no insurance or money)
- hospital discharge planner
- hospital-based home health agencies
- the school of nursing at a local community college
- college employment offices
- hospices (call the National Hospice Organization)
- nurses' registries
- Catholic Charities, Jewish Family Services, and other faith-based groups
- the American Red Cross
- churches, synagogues, mosques
- a nearby nursing home employee who seeks part-time work
- an adult relative whom you would pay a fair hourly wage for services

Types of Health Care Professionals

Registered Nurse (RN)—has at least 2 years of school training and is licensed by the state Board of Nursing Examiners

Licensed Practical Nurse (LPN)—has finished a one-year course of study and is licensed by the state Board of Licensed Vocational Nurses

Certified Nurses Aide (CNA)—has finished 70 hours of classes and 50 hours of clinical practice in a nursing center setting; must pass a test and register with the State Board of Nursing

Home Health Aide—is screened on the basis of work experience; training and requirements differ from state to state

Someone who is taking classes or is in a training program that leads to one of the above professions might be able to help with care.

Tax Rules You Must Follow If You Hire Privately

- If you paid more than $1,400 in 2005 or $1,500 in 2006, you are required to pay Medicare and Social Security tax.

- You may use federal income tax return Form 1040 to pay the Social Security, Medicare, and Federal Unemployment (FUTA) taxes. Ask the Internal Revenue Service for the *Household Employer's Tax Guide.*

- For tax information, call the Social Security office. Look in the front of your phone book under State Government.

How to Screen a Personal Hire

- Check licenses, training, experience, and references.
- Be sure the person who is applying for hire has malpractice or liability insurance.
- Run a criminal background check and a driving record check (through a private investigator). Also, ask to see the person's insurance card.
- Find out if the person has a special skill (for example, working with care receivers who have multiple sclerosis or other neurological disorders).
- Decide whether the person is someone who can meet the emotional needs of the person in your care.
- Consider his or her personal habits.
- Find out if he or she is a smoker or nonsmoker.

You can hire a private investigator to look at public records and check on education and licenses, driving history, and previous employers. This service can be obtained anywhere in the country.

Questions to Ask of the Applicant's References:

When someone is going to be hired, ask for the names of people who can tell you about this person's work and personal habits. Here are some questions you can ask:

- How long have you known this person?

- Did this person work for you?

- Is this person reliable, on time for work, patient, able to adjust as things change, able to be trusted, and polite?

- How does this person handle disagreements and emergencies?

- How well does this person follow directions, respond to requests, and take advice?

Perform All Caregiving Duties Yourself

If you decide to provide all the caregiving yourself, you can receive training at the following places:

- social service agencies

- hospitals

- community schools

- the American Red Cross

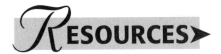

RESOURCES➤

Eldercare Locator
(800) 677-1116
www.eldercare.gov
Provides information about local support resources providing services to the elderly.

Family Caregiver Alliance
690 Market Street, Suite 600
San Francisco, CA 94104
(800) 445-8106; 415-434-3388 Fax: (415) 434-3508
www.caregiver.org
E-mail: info@caregiver.org
Resource center for caregivers of people with chronic disabling conditions. The Web site provides information on services and programs in education, research, and advocacy.

National Family Caregivers Association
10400 Connecticut Avenue, Suite 500
Kensington, MD 20895-3944
(800) 896-3650; (301) 942-6430
www.thefamilycaregiver.org
Email: info@thefamilycaregiver.org
The Association supports, empowers, educates, and speaks up for more than 50 million Americans who care for a chronically ill, aged, or disabled person.

Home Care Agencies/Hiring Help

The Center for Applied Gerontology, Council for Jewish Elderly
3003 W. Touhy Avenue
Chicago, IL 60645.
(773) 508-1000
E-mail: cag@cje.net
www.cje.net/professional/cag_orderform_2.pdf
Offers a 32-page pamphlet "Someone Who Cares: A Guide to Hiring an In-Home Caregiver." $9.95 plus $3.50 shipping and handling.

National Association for Home Care
228 Seventh Street, SE
Washington, DC 20003
(202) 547-7424
www.nahc.org
Provides referrals to state associations, which can refer callers to local agencies. Offers publications, including the free pamphlet "How to Choose a Home Care Agency: A Consumer's Guide." Information on finding help, interviewing, reference checking, training, being a good manager, maintaining a good working and personal relationship, problems that might arise and how best to solve them, service dogs, assistive technology, and tax responsibilities. Contains sample forms and letters.

Publications

Avoiding Attendants from Hell: A Practical Guide to Finding, Hiring and Keeping Personal Care Attendants by June Price; Science & Humanities Press.

Managing Personal Assistants: A Consumer Guide, published by Paralyzed Veterans of America. To purchase a copy call (888) 860-7244, or download online at www.pva.org/cgi-bin/pvastore/products.cgi?id=2

If you don't have access to the Internet, ask your local library to help you locate a Web site.

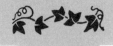

Paying for Care

Paying for Care

$\mathcal{Y}$ou can look to many sources for help in paying for care. Some are public, while others are private or volunteer. The most common ways to pay for home care are as follows:

- *personal and family resources*

- *private insurance*

- *Medicare, Medicaid, Department of Veterans Affairs, and Title programs*

- *community-based services*

Assessment of Financial Resources

First, complete a personal financial resources assessment by doing the following:

- Look at current assets, where the person's income comes from, and insurance entitlements.

- Prepare a budget and figure out what the person's future income might be from all sources.

- Confirm the qualifications, retirement benefits, and Social Security status of the person in your care.

- Figure as closely as possible the expenses of professional care and equipment. Include any medical procedures likely to be needed.

- Check on the person's personal tax status and find out what care items and expenses are deductible.

- Find out if the person's health insurance or employer's workers' compensation policy has home health care benefits.

- Figure out how much money the person will need.

 Think about making the person in your care a "dependent" and thus be able to transfer medical expenses to a taxpayer who can make use of medical deductions.

Public Pay Programs

Medicare

Medicare is a federal health insurance program. It provides health care benefits to all Americans 65 and older and to those who have been determined to be "disabled" according to the Social Security Administration. There are constant changes in Medicare policies, requirements, and forms. Therefore, it is always best to get the most current information on benefits by calling the Medicare Hotline (p. 106) or your hospital's social worker.

Things That Affect Medicare Eligibility

Whether the Person Is Homebound—Medicare will pay for certain home health care services only if the person is confined to the home and requires part-time skilled (nursing) services or therapy. Medicare does not cover ongoing custodial (maintenance) care. "Confined to home" does not mean bedridden. It means that a person cannot leave home except for medical care and requires help to get there. (Brief absences from the home do not affect eligibility.)

In order for treatments, services, and supplies to be paid, they must be ordered by a doctor. They must also be provided by a home health agency certified by Medicare and the state health department.

Whether Care Is Intermittent (periodic)—In order to be covered, skilled services are required. Medicare is not designed to meet chronic ongoing needs that are considered "custodial" rather than "skilled."

Medicare Generally Pays for the Following:

- almost all costs of skilled care, such as doctors, nurses, and specialists
- various types of therapy—occupational, physical, speech-language
- home health services
- medical supplies and equipment
- personal care by home health aides (such as bathing, dressing, fixing meals, even light housekeeping and counseling) after discharge from a hospital or nursing home

Medicare Part D—Prescription Drug Plan

Beginning January 1, 2006, Medicare will cover prescription drugs. There are two basic ways to sign up for this coverage. If you have traditional Medicare (Part A for hospital services and Part B for doctor and outpatient health-care providers), you may sign up for a stand-alone Medicare Part D prescription drug plan. You can also choose a managed care plan under Medicare Advantage. These plans restrict you to only the doctors on the managed-care provider's list. They also have a prescription drug plan. All plans are from private companies that have been approved by Medicare (*see Resources*, p. 106).

Help is available to pay for copayments and premiums for those whose incomes are low enough to be eligible. A person must apply to the Social Security Administration for financial assistance.

Phrases like "intermittent care," "skilled care," and "homebound" are not precisely defined. They are different from region to region, and the type and availability of coverage by Medicare may be different as well.

Services NOT covered by Medicare

Full-time nursing care at home, drugs, meals delivered to the home, homemaker chore services *not* related to care, and personal care services are usually not covered by Medicare.

 A caregiver who has power of attorney for a person on Medicare (the beneficiary) must send written permission to the person's Medicare Part B carrier. Send a letter with the person's name, number, signature, and a statement that the caregiver can act on behalf of the beneficiary. The form must list start and end dates.

If there is a dispute about a repayment from Medicare, a review may be requested by filing a claim with the Medicare carrier.

Medicare Part B Insurance

Medicare Part B insurance costs $88.50 per month (2006) and $93.50 (2007) offers extra benefits to basic Medicare coverage. It pays for tests, doctor's office visits, lab services, and home health care. A $124 deductible applies.

Medicare Supplemental Insurance (Medigap)

To pay for benefits not covered by Medicare, this private health insurance option is available. It pays for noncovered services only—for example, hospital deductibles, doctor copayments, and eyeglasses—but does not cover long-term care services. Coverage depends on the plan you buy.

For anyone who has Medicare HMO coverage, Medigap insurance may not be necessary because those individuals only make a small copayment but do not pay a deductible for doctor's visits.

> **NOTE** It is illegal for an insurance company or agent to sell you a second Medigap policy unless you put in writing that you intend to end the Medigap policy you have. The federal toll-free telephone number for filing complaints is (800) 638-6833.

Medicaid

Medicaid pays for the medical care of low-income elderly persons or those whose assets have been used up while paying for their own care. Eligibility depends on monthly income limits and personal assets. Coverage includes nursing facilities, assisted living, foster care, and certain types of home care. Each state runs its own Medicaid program, and so eligibility and coverage can vary. Some states have set up Medicaid Waiver programs, which pay for home and community-based services that would otherwise only be paid if one were in a nursing home.

Common Aspects of Medicaid

- Recipients must be financially and medically in need.

- For recipients who are terminally ill, benefits go on for as long as they are ill. However, care must be provided by an agency with hospice certification and Medicaid certification.

- Payments are made directly to providers of services.

- Long-term-care costs are paid for those not covered by insurance and for patients whose finances have run out.

- Payments to foster care homes and retirement communities are not covered (except in some cases by Medicaid waiver).

- Home health care services, medical supplies, and equipment are covered.

- Eligibility is based on a person's income and assets.

- People with disabilities who are eligible for state public assistance are eligible for Medicaid.

- People with disabilities eligible for Supplemental Social Security (SSI) are eligible for Medicaid.

- In many states, there are laws (called spousal impoverishment laws) that protect a portion of the estate and assets for the healthy spouse. These come into play after other monies have been "spent down" for the care of the ill spouse.

To find out what the benefits are, contact the local Social Security office, city or county public assistance office, or the Area Agency on Aging.

Services NOT covered by Medicaid

As a rule, Medicare, Medicaid, and private insurance do not cover many in-home services because they are not medical services. However, some community services may be called on to fill the gap for free or on a subsidized (public funding) basis. The following services usually are not covered but might be available locally free of charge:

- adult day care

- alcohol and drug programs

- case management

- household chore services

- neighborhood and local meal services, such as Meals on Wheels

- consumer protection

- transportation

- emergency response systems (which provide contact by phone or electronic device to police and rescue services)

- emergency assistance for food, clothing, or shelter

- friendly visitors (volunteers who stop by to write letters or run errands)

- services and equipment for those who have disabilities

- homemaker services

- legal and financial services

- mental health services

- respite care

- senior centers

- support groups (which will send materials if you write to them)

- telephone reassurance (volunteers who make calls to or receive calls from those who are elderly or living alone)

 The U.S. Congress and the Administration made major changes to Medicare and Medicaid, which will affect payment for long-term care. As these changes are put into effect, they are posted on the Web site of the Center for Medicare and Medicaid Services (CMS): www.cms.gov

Department of Veterans Affairs Benefits

Veterans generally qualify for health services in the home if a disability is service related. Even if a disability is not service related, other benefits may be available based on income qualifications. Some states have special programs only for veterans who live in that state. Some Veterans Hospitals have programs to deliver home health care services. Contact the nearest Veterans Affairs office or veterans group in your area.

Older Americans Act and Social Services Block Grant

Some agencies that provide support services get funding under this program. Services available may include the following:

- case management and assessment
- household chore services (minor household repairs, cleaning, yard work)
- companion services
- community meals
- home-delivered hot meals (Meals on Wheels) once or twice a day
- homemaker services
- transportation

Private Pay Long-Term-Care Insurance

Generally, private insurance programs do not cover long-term care. In many cases, home care reimbursement is severely restricted or prohibited. Policies must be examined closely. Before buying long-term care insurance, seek the best, most knowledgeable help available on the subject (for example, consult a hospital discharge planner or the Area Agency on Aging). Seek agents who represent reliable companies and have a reputation for honesty. The lack of uniformity in long-term care policies makes it hard to compare them.

- Policies vary greatly so don't assume one is like another you are familiar with.

- It's important to read the fine print.

- Such policies should not be considered an option for anyone over 79.

- Coverage is often limited to Medicare-certified nursing homes.

- Sometimes benefits are provided for hospice care for the terminally ill.

- Benefits are usually $50–$200 per day.

- A typical policy for a healthy 65-year-old costs about $3,000 per year.

- Long-term-care insurance should be purchased before age 60, when premiums are relatively low.

- The best companies are those that offer direct cash for home care instead of reimbursement (so payment can be used for a family caregiver).

- It is important to buy what you can comfortably afford.

Long-term-care insurance has two parts:

- In-home care benefits, which usually pay $100 per day for personal and domestic chores provided by a licensed home health agency.

- Nursing home benefits of approximately $200 a day.

To activate a policy, the policy holder must get confirmation from a doctor that he or she has lost the ability to do two or more of the following: bathing, eating, dressing, moving without falling, going to the toilet, and moving

Checklist **Long-Term-Care Insurance Policies**

✓ Look for an insurer that is top rated by Moody's Investors Service, A.M. Best Company, or Standard & Poor's Corporation.

✓ Find out how long the company has been in business and check the Better Business Bureau or the state's Insurance Division for complaints.

✓ Take someone with you when you meet the agent.

✓ Never pay cash to an agent. The payment should be made by check written to the insurance company and be sure the agent gives you a signed and dated receipt when the policy is delivered.

✓ Find premiums that do not exceed 5–6% of the covered individual's income.

✓ Ask for an "Outline of Coverage" which the law requires the insurance company to provide even if you do not want to fill out an application for insurance. Use this outline to compare policies.

✓ Understand how and when you can contact the care manager.

✓ Look for a policy that pays for care at home, in any adult foster care home, assisted living facility, and nursing home (not just one that is Medicare certified).

✓ Avoid policies that cover only skilled care. Look for policies that allow respite care and adult day care.

✓ Find out when the insurance pays for home custodial care or hospice care.

✓ Find out if previous hospitalization, a nursing home stay, or other restrictive eligibility criteria are required.

✓ Be sure that benefits will increase with inflation (5% each year).

✓ Make sure that benefits last at least three years if you don't buy lifetime benefits.

✓ Find out if some coverage is provided if the policy lapses and what conditions must be met before benefits can be started.

✓ Make sure the policy is guaranteed renewable regardless of age.

✓ Get several proposals before making a decision.

from a bed to a chair. The insurance company will send its representative to confirm the diagnosis. Homemaker benefits usually do not go into effect until 60 to 100 days after a hospital stay, and strict criteria must be met before in-home help is provided.

Consider Long-Term-Care Insurance If:

- Personal assets exceed $100,000 for a couple or $50,000 for a single person and need to be protected.

- The assets cannot be transferred.

- There is a family history of frail-elderly.

- No one will be available to care for the person.

 NOTE Many states license individuals to offer analysis of insurance coverage for a fee. In some states if a person has a license to sell and a license to counsel, he or she can only perform one of those services for a specific client. Check your state department of insurance for information about insurance counselors.

Health Maintenance Organizations (HMOs)

Health Maintenance Organizations are prepaid health insurance plans that give complete medical coverage for a fixed premium. Knowing whether an HMO is right for the person in your care requires careful study.

Types of HMOs

There are three types of HMOs:

IPA (Individual Practice Associations) Plans—A patient chooses a doctor from a primary care physician list.

POS (Point of Service) Plans—For an extra fee a patient can visit a doctor outside of the network list.

Group Model HMOs—A patient must go to a clinic for treatment.

Remember, HMOs receive the same fees to treat a healthy person as a person with a chronic disease. For some patients with long-term or chronic illness, HMOs may not be a good choice. A patient who has a long-established relationship with a specialist who is not a member of the HMO's network list may not be able to continue to see that specialist.

 If a Medicare health plan is not meeting the needs of the person in your care, it is not difficult to switch to another plan or to a fee-for-service program.

How To Determine If an HMO Is Right for Your Survivor

- Ask if the doctor or specialist the person is now seeing is in the HMO network.

- Understand the person's medical needs—for special equipment, drugs, and help with activities. Determine if these needs are covered.

- Find out if the HMO is used to dealing with the illness the person has.

- Determine the specific services offered for this type of illness.

- Ask who decides what is medically necessary.

- Ask if there is a special Plan of Care for the illness.

- Ask if the person will get the *best* drugs for the condition or if generic substitutes will be offered.

- Ask how many people with this type of illness are under the plan in your area.

- Verify that the patient may see the specialists listed in the directory.

- Ask if the plan allows visits to specialists without a primary care doctor's referral.

- If a referral is required, find out how long it lasts and if a new referral is required for every visit.

- Ask what percentage of doctors on the list are board certified (have passed a special test given by the board of their specialty).

- Ask if the doctor has a financial incentive to do tests or to keep the patient from having tests or seeing a specialist.

- Ask if the plan covers visits to doctors outside the plan's referral list. (Out-of-network coverage may be limited to a certain dollar amount.)

- Ask how many doctors in the HMO specialize in geriatric care.

- If the person in your care must travel to a specific locale for extended stays, be sure the HMO allows visits to a different HMO there.

- Ask how the person will be charged if an emergency room visit is needed while traveling.

- Ask about the process for appealing a medical decision.

- Once you have decided on an HMO, get confirmation in writing regarding the items or services that are most important to the person in your care.

To find out how many patient complaints were registered against an HMO, call your state insurance commissioner in the phone book under State Government.

How to Appeal an HMO's Decision Regarding a Medical Procedure, Prescription, or Specialist Referral

When a treatment is denied, the goal is to reverse the denial as quickly as possible. Remember that the HMO can prolong a case in court, so the goal is to resolve the case without litigation.

- Call the HMO and ask for a copy of its formal appeals process. (Federal law requires HMOs to have such a process.)

- Make detailed notes of all conversations with the HMO; include the date and the staff person's name.

- Determine exactly why the HMO refused to cover the treatment.

- Ask the HMO clerk for an explanation; if the matter is not resolved, ask for the HMO medical director's explanation of denial of treatment.

- If you still feel the situation is not resolved, start a written appeal process.

- Ask the doctor for a written explanation why treatment is medically necessary (also ask the specialists you have visited for a letter of support.)

- Save all bills related to the problem.

- For consumer advice or support for the appeal, call the state insurance department, state health department, advocacy group for the disease, or local Area Agency on Aging.

> *Tip* The clerk at the other end of the line is a person too, and being courteous always gets a better response than being viewed as irrational or disrespectful.

Community-Based Services

Many services are provided free by local or community groups. The groups are sometimes repaid by state, local, and federal governments, but often volunteers provide meals and social and health care services.

These services can sometimes make it possible for a person to stay at home and maintain independence.

Typical Services

Community-based services include the following:

Adult Day Care Centers, which provide services ranging from health assessment to social programs that help people with dementia or those at risk for nursing home placement.

Nutrition Sites, which serve meals in settings such as senior centers, housing projects, faith-based centers, and schools and sometimes provide transportation.

Meals on Wheels, which brings healthful food to the home.

Senior Centers, which offer a place to socialize and eat. (Often a hot meal at noontime on weekdays is the only one served.)

Transportation is offered by hospitals, nursing homes, local governments, and religious, civic, or other groups. Out-of-pocket costs vary and fees are set on a sliding scale based on ability to pay.

Do These Services Meet Your Needs?

For whatever need you have, there is most likely a program in your area. Here are some things to think about:

- Is the person the right age and income level to be eligible for the program?
- Is it necessary for the person to belong to a certain organization to be eligible?
- Is there a limit to how many times the person can use the services of the organization?

Where to Check

- local agencies (Catholic Charities, United Way, Jewish Family and Child Services, Lutheran Family Services)
- local churches, parishes, or congregations
- the government blue book pages under public service listings
- city or county public assistance offices
- rural areas (call the health agency in the county seat)
- personal doctor
- family services department
- hospital discharge planner or social worker
- insurance company
- local Area Agency on Aging
- previous or current employer (may have benefits)
- public health department
- Social Security office
- state insurance commission
- state or local ombudsman

The Area Agency on Aging can help find services in the community. It will know whether chore services, home-delivered meals, friendly visitors, and telephone reassurance are free of charge or are provided on a sliding scale.

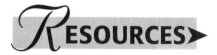

RESOURCES

AARP
601 E. Street, NW
Washington, D.C. 20049
(800) 424-3410
www.aarp.org
Provides information on Medicare beneficiaries.

Centers for Medicare and Medicaid Services
7500 Security Boulevard
Baltimore, MD 21244-1850
(800) MEDICARE (633-4227) Medicare Hotline
www.cms.gov
www.medicare.gov
Federal agency that administers the Medicare and Medicaid programs, including hospice benefits.

National Association of Professional Geriatric Care Managers
1604 N. Country Club Road
Tucson, AZ 85716
(520) 881-8008
www.caremanager.org
Their Web site provides a free list of care managers in your state.

The National Council on the Aging
300 D Street SW, Suite 801
Washington, D.C. 20024
(202) 479-1200
www.ncoa.org
Provides a link to benefits (www.benefitscheckup.org) that helps seniors find state and federal benefits programs.

If you don't have access to the Internet, ask your local library to help you locate a Web site.

Preparing the Home

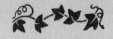

Preparing the Home

It may be necessary to make some changes to your home. Most families find that they do not have to redesign their home. It is important, however, to look at one's home with an eye toward saving energy, making work easier to do, and making the home more accessible (easier for the person in your care to use). It is better to make changes sooner rather than later.

We believe it is important for our readers to be aware of the "ideal" as they plan the changes they will make. If you are thinking of buying a new home, use these guidelines to help choose the right home that will meet future needs.

Adapting for Safety, Accessibility, and Comfort

The main goal in any home is safety. You and the person in your care need to take a close look at your home. You may also want to ask the advice of a friend or relative.

> **NOTE** Leave a blanket, pillow, and phone on the floor; however, not in the flow of foot traffic. In case of a fall, the person in your care can stay warm and call for help.

As you plan for safety in the home, consider what you need now and what you will need in the future. For example, furniture that works well now may need to be changed or replaced later when the person can no longer get up from low seats. Your main goal is to make the home as safe as possible.

As you make changes to the home, don't forget your own comfort and ease. Making life easier for yourself means you will have more time to provide care or to rest. In the long run, this will improve the overall setting for care.

The Home Environment

The ideal home for a survivor is on one level (ground floor). Having more than one floor is all right only if there is an elevator or another approved lift device, or if the person in your care does not need to go to the second floor. The ideal care home is laid out in such a way that the caregiver and the person in care can see each other from other rooms.

Safety

For the safest home, follow as many of these steps as possible:

- Remove all furniture that is not needed.

- Place the remaining furniture so that there is enough space for a walker or wheelchair. This will avoid the need for a person who is elderly or disabled to move around coffee tables and other barriers. Move any low tables that are in the way.

- Once the person in your care has gotten used to where the furniture is, do not change it.

- Make sure furniture will not move if leaned on.

- Ensure that the armrests of a favorite chair are long enough to help the person get up and down.

- Modify or cushion sharp corners on furniture, cabinets, and vanities.

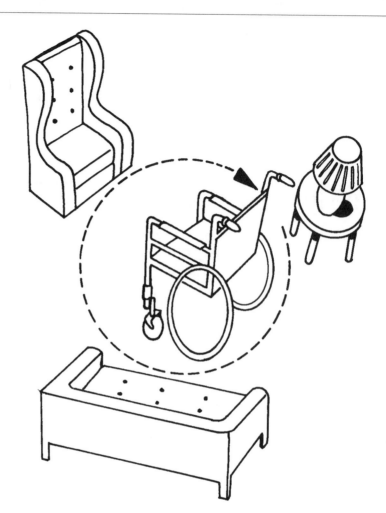

▶ *To accommodate a wheelchair, arrange furniture 5¹/₂ feet apart.*

- Make chair seats 20″ high. (Wood blocks or a wooden platform can be placed under large, heavy furniture to raise it to this level.)

- Have a carpenter put railings in places where a person might need extra support. (Using a carpenter can ensure that railings will bear a person's full weight and will not give way.)

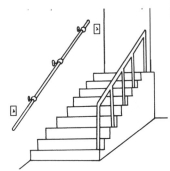

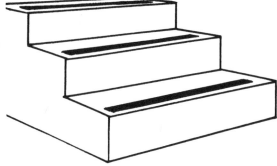

▶ *Place nonskid tape on the edges of steps.*

▲ *Always provide railings along stairways. When possible, extend the handrail past the bottom and top step.*

- Place masking or colored tape on glass doors and picture windows.

- Use automatic night-lights in the rooms used by the person in your care.

- Clear fire-escape routes.

- Put smoke alarms on every floor and outside every bedroom.

- Place a fire extinguisher in the kitchen.

- Consider the need for monitors and intercoms.

- Place nonskid tape on the edges of stairs. (Consider painting the edge of the first and last step a different color from the floor.)

- Thin-piled carpet is easier to walk on than thick pile. Avoid "busy" patterns.

NOTE ▶ For a safer home setting for a person with a respiratory (breathing) condition such as asthma, emphysema, or chronic bronchitis, avoid the following:

- rugs
- belt-type humidifiers
- overstuffed furniture
- books and book shelves
- pets and stuffed toys
- pleated lampshades
- dirty heat ducts and air filters
- tobacco smoke
- wool blankets and clothing

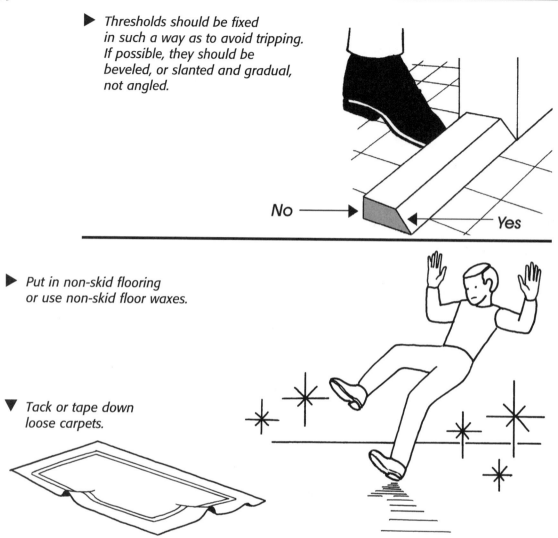

▶ Thresholds should be fixed in such a way as to avoid tripping. If possible, they should be beveled, or slanted and gradual, not angled.

No → ← Yes

▶ Put in non-skid flooring or use non-skid floor waxes.

▼ Tack or tape down loose carpets.

- Be sure stairs have an even surface with no metal strips or rubber mats that can cause tripping.

- Remove anything that might lead to tripping.

- Secure electrical and telephone cords to walls.

- Adjust or remove rapidly closing doors.

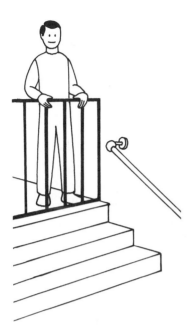

▲ *A safety gate at the top of stairs can prevent falls.*

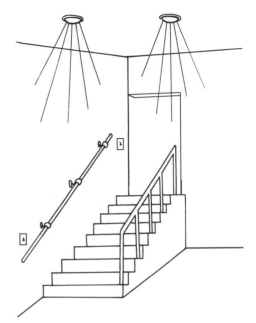

▲ *Be sure steps are well lighted with light switches at both the top and bottom of the stairs.*

- Place protective screens on fireplaces.

- Cover exposed hot water pipes.

- Provide plenty of indirect no-glare lighting.

- Place light switches next to room entrances so the lights can be turned on before entering a room. Consider "clap-on" lamps beside the bed.

- Use 100–200 watt lightbulbs for close-up activities (but make sure lamps can handle the extra wattage).

NOTE Contrasting colors play a big part in seeing well. As much as possible, the color of furniture, toilet seats, counters, etc., should be different from the floor color.

- Plan for extra outdoor lighting for good nighttime visibility, especially on stairs and walkways.

- If possible, install a carbon monoxide (CO) detector that sounds an alarm when dangerous levels of CO are reached. Call the **American Lung Association** at 1-800-LUNG USA for details.

- Develop an emergency evacuation plan in case of fire.

> **NOTE** If the person in your care is on life-support equipment, install a backup electrical system and have a plan of action if the power goes out.

Comfort and Convenience

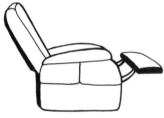

- For persons who are frail or wheelchair-bound, put in automatic door openers.

- For a person with a wheelchair or a walker, allow at least 18″ to 24″ clearance from the door on landings.

- Plan to leave enough space (a minimum of 32″ clear) for moving a hospital bed and wheelchair through doorways.

▲ *Think about getting a power-assisted recliner that allows the power-assist feature to be turned off.*

▶ *Install entry ramps. Rails can be added for more safety. Ramps should not rise more than 1″ per foot, and should be 30–40″ wide.*

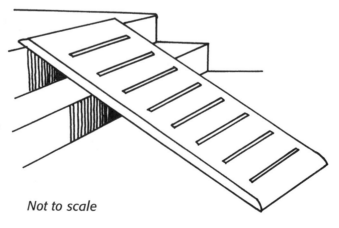

Not to scale

> **NOTE** If you are redoing a two-story house or building a new one, have the contractor frame in the shell of the elevator and then add the elevator unit later if needed. Use the space as a closet now.

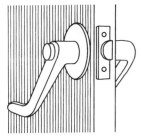

▲ *Lever handle*

- To widen doorways, remove the molding and replace regular door hinges with offset hinges. Whenever possible, remove doors.

- Install lever handles on all doors.

- If a person who is disabled must be moved from one story to another, install a stair elevator.

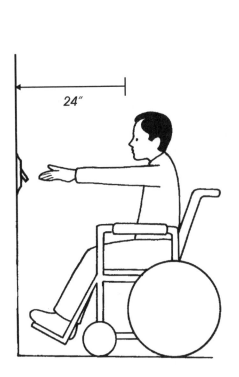

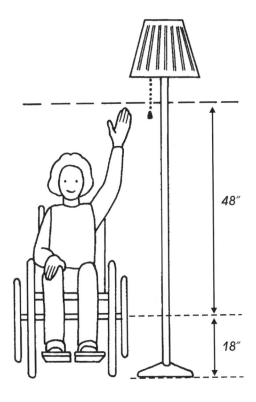

▲ *A person can reach forward about 24" from a seated position. Between 18" and 48" from the floor is the ideal position for light switches, telephones, and mailboxes.*

The Bathroom

Many accidents happen in bathrooms, so check the safety of the bathroom that you will use for home care.

Safety

▶ Install grab bars beside and in back of the toilet, along the edge of the sink, and in the tub and shower according to the needs of each person.

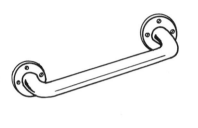

▶ Five-inch door pulls or utility handles can be put on door frames and window sills.

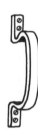

- Cover all sharp edges with rubber cushioning.

- Install lights in medicine cabinets so mistakes are not made when taking medicine.

- Remove locks on bathroom doors.

- Use nonskid safety strips or a nonslip bath mat in the tub or shower.

- Consider installing a grab rail on the edge of the vanity. (Do not use a towel bar.)

- Remove glass shower doors or replace them with un-breakable plastic.

- Use only electrical appliances with a ground fault interrupted (GFI) feature.

- Install GFI electrical outlets.

- Set the hot water thermostat below 120° F.

- Use faucets that mix hot and cold water, or paint hot water knobs and faucets red.

- Insulate hot water pipes to prevent burns.

- Install toilet guard rails or provide a portable toilet seat with built-in rails. (📖 See *Equipment and Supplies*, p. 136.)

Comfort and Convenience

- If possible, have the bathroom in a straight path from the bedroom of the person in your care.

- Install a ceiling heat lamp.

- Place a telephone near the toilet.

- Provide soap-on-a-rope or put a bar of soap in the toe of a nylon stocking and tie it to the grab bar.

- Place toilet paper within easy reach.

- Try to provide enough space for two people at the bathroom sink.

- If possible, have the sink 32″ to 34″ from the floor.

- Use levers instead of handles on the faucets.

- Provide a raised (elevated) toilet seat.

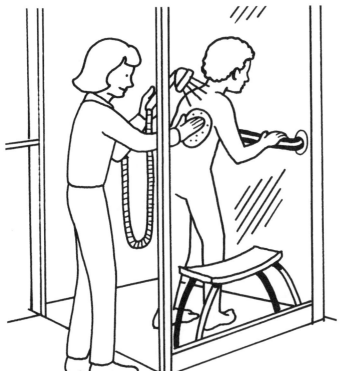

◀ *If possible, have a shower stall that is large enough for two people. Use a hand-held shower head with a very long hose and adjustable jet stream. Put a tub seat or bench in the shower stall.*

The Kitchen

Many of the following suggestions are made to fit the needs of people who are disabled who are able to help in the kitchen.

Safety

- Use an electric teakettle.
- Set the water-heater temperature at 120° F.
- Use a single lever faucet that can balance water temperature.
- Provide an area away from the knife drawer and the stove where the person in your care can help prepare food.
- Use a microwave oven whenever possible (but not if a person with a pacemaker is present).

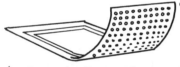

- Ask the gas company to modify your stove to provide a gas odor strong enough to alert you if the pilot light goes out.

▲ *Cover the floor with a nonslip surface or use a nonskid mat near the sink, where it may be wet.*

- If possible, have the range controls on the front of the stove.
- Provide a step stool, never a chair, to reach high shelves.

Comfort and Convenience

- Use adjustable-height chairs with locking casters.
- Install a Lazy Susan (swivel plate) in corner cabinets.
- Rearrange cabinets to reduce bending and reaching.
- Install a storage wall rather than upper cabinets.
- For easy access, replace drawer knobs with handles.

▶ *Use "reachers"—devices for reaching objects in high or low places without stretching, bending, or standing on a stool.*

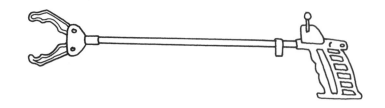

▶ *A cutting board placed over a drawer provides an easy-to-reach surface for a person in a wheelchair.*

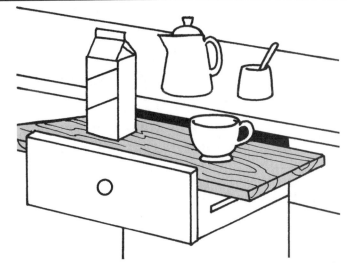

- To reduce back strain from reaching dishes, place a wire rack on the counter.

- Adapt one counter for wheelchair access as pictured above.

- Remove doors under the sink to accommodate a wheelchair; also insulate exposed pipes.

- Create different counter heights by installing folding or pullout surfaces.

- When bending is difficult, consider a wall oven.

- Use drawer suspension systems for heavy drawers.

- Install pullout shelves in cabinets.

- If possible, use a refrigerator that has the freezer on the bottom.

- Prop the front of the refrigerator so that the door closes automatically. (If necessary, reverse the way the door swings.)

The Bedroom

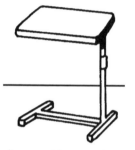

▲ *Provide an adjustable over-the-bed table like the ones used to serve meals in hospital rooms.*

Ideally provide three bedrooms—one for the person in care, one for yourself, and one for the home health aide. Also—

- Install a monitor to listen to activity in the room of the person in your care. (Some are inexpensive and portable.)

- Make the bedroom bright and cheerful.

- Make sure adequate heat (65° F at night) and fresh air are available.

- Provide a firm mattress.

- Provide TV and radio.

- Consider a fish aquarium for distraction and relaxation.

- Use disposable pads to protect furniture.

- Install room-darkening blinds or shades.

- Place closet rods 48″ from the floor.

- Provide a chair for dressing.

- Keep a flashlight at the bedside table.

- Provide a bedside commode with a 4″ foam pad on the seat for comfort.

- Hang a bulletin board with pictures of family and friends where it can be easily seen.

- Provide a sturdy chair or table next to the bed for help getting in and out of bed.

- Make the bed 22″ high and stabilize it against a wall. Or use a bed with wheels that can be locked. This will allow the person who uses it to get up and down safely.

- Use blocks to raise a bed's height, but be sure to stabilize them carefully.

▶ *Bedside commode and bed with trapeze bar*

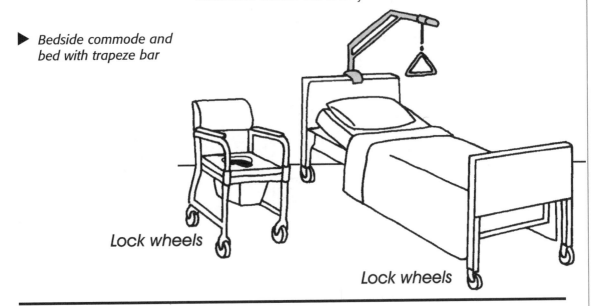

Lock wheels

Lock wheels

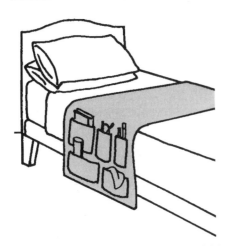

▲ *Make a bed organizer to hold facial tissues, lotion, and other items needed at the bedside. Do this by attaching pockets to a large piece of fabric spread across the bed.*

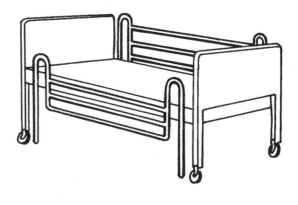

▲ *If all the care is at the bedside, consider a hospital bed. This will be helpful for both you and the person in your care.*

The Telephone

Contact your local phone company's special-needs department or visit a store that sells phones and accessories to inquire about—

- increasing the number size on your phone dial for improved visibility and ease of use

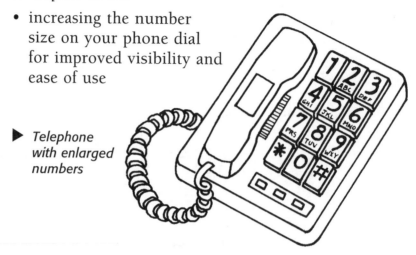

▶ *Telephone with enlarged numbers*

- a phone cradle

- step-by-step, large-size instructions for using the phone

- amplified handsets

- signal devices, such as lights that flash when a call is coming in

- TTY (text telephone yoke), a device for people with hearing loss

- a portable phone

- speed-dial buttons with names or pictures of friends and family instead of numbers

- a one-line phone that automatically connects to a pre-set number when the button is pressed

- a list of emergency numbers and medicines beside the telephone (📖 See *Setting Up a Plan of Care,* p. 162, for a sample)

- clear instructions on how to direct emergency personnel to the street address of the house

- a personal emergency response system to signal a friend or emergency service

 NOTE Some communities provide a free telephone reassurance service. TRS will make a brief, daily telephone call to persons who are elderly or disabled to reassure them and to share crime prevention information. Call your local police department.

Outdoor Areas

Safe outdoor areas are important. Outdoor safety features should include:

- ramps for access on uneven ground

- a deck with a sturdy railing

- outside doors that are locked or have alarms

- a hidden key outside

- enough light to see walkways at night

- nonslip step surfaces in good repair

- stair handrails fastened to their fittings

- step edges marked with reflective paint

In addition, unplug or remove power tools.

Additional Considerations

It is important to find out how many levels of living space there are inside and outside your home. Note any possible access problems. Canes, crutches, and walkers need a certain amount of open space for moving around and turning. Wheelchairs and scooters require a wide turning area.

You and the person in your care need to think about your activities at home. Ask who, what, where, when, why, and how about everything you do. Who can help with what specific jobs? What jobs can you get rid of or make simpler? Would you be more comfortable doing the job somewhere else? Can you make the home more pleasant? In terms of work centers, plan where you can sit for each of your activities so that everything you need is at hand. Ask for input from everyone in the family. Making work simpler will help the stroke survivor and can save time as well.

If Changes Are Needed

Changing certain things can increase safety, accessibility, and comfort for everyone. But before making major changes to the home, ask a doctor for a referral to an occupational therapist (OT) for a home visit. An OT can recommend ways to keep the stroke survivor as independent as possible, ensure safety, and reduce the physical strain on the caregiver. Ramps, wider doorways, and repairs in the kitchen and bath can often solve accessibility problems. Not all changes are major expenses.

Almost any equipment or installation required by a disability can be tax deductible, within IRS rules and guidelines.

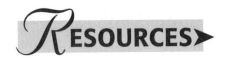

ESOURCES

Check with local police to find out if they manage a **Senior Locks Program**. This is a program whereby homeowners 55 and older who meet federal income guidelines can have deadbolt locks and other security devices installed at no charge.

AARP
601 E Street, NW
Washington, DC 20049
(800) 424-3410
www.aarp.org
Call or write for the booklet The Do-Able, Renewable Home. *Members can receive one copy at no charge.*

Center for Universal Design
North Carolina State University
Box 8613
Raleigh, NC 27695-8613
(919) 515-3082 (V/TTY) Fax (919) 515-3023
(800) 647-6777
www.design.ncsu.edu\cud
E-mail: cud@ncsu.edu
Established to improve the quality and availability of housing for people with disabilities. Services include information, referral service, training and education, technical design assistance, and publications.

Metropolitan Center for Independent Living, Inc. (MCIL)
1600 University Avenue West, Suite 16
St. Paul, MN 55104-3825
(651) 603-2029
www.wheelchairramp.org
E-mail: jimwi@mcil-mn.org
Web site features How to Build Wheelchair Ramps for Homes, *an online manual for the design and construction of wheelchair ramps.*

National Association of Home Builders Research Center
(800) 638-8556; (301) 249-4000
www.nahbrc.org
Call for its book A Comprehensive Approach to Retrofit-ting Houses for a Lifetime, *$15 plus postage and handling.*

National Institute for Rehabilitation Engineering
P.O. Box 1088
Hewett, NJ 07421
(800) 736-2216; (973) 853-6585 Fax (928) 832-2894
www.theoffice.net/nire
E-mail: nire@theoffice.net

Paralyzed Veterans of America
801 18th Street NW
Washington, DC 20006-3517
Tel: 1-800-424-8200
www.pva.org
Not just for veterans, not just for paralysis. Ask for the Architecture Program.

If you don't have access to the Internet, ask your local library to help you locate a Web site.

Equipment and Supplies

Equipment and Supplies

*T*o provide proper at-home care, you will need certain supplies. There are two types:

- *general medical supplies*
- *durable medical equipment*

Before buying anything or signing a rental contract, ask your doctor, physical or occupational therapist, or nurse. Salespeople may not be trained to assess what the person in your care may need. Occupational therapists can advise you on low-cost substitutes for expensive equipment. With the proper doctor's orders (referrals) and documentation, some equipment is covered by Medicare or private insurance. Get in touch with your insurance carrier to see if what you need is covered and follow the company's rules for getting approval before buying.

Where to Buy Needed Supplies

Buy medical equipment and supplies from dealers that are well established and that are well known for good service. Be sure to get advice about where to buy from your health care professionals or hospital discharge planner. To compare prices, use the chart on page 145.

Look in the Yellow Pages under Surgical Appliances, Physicians and Surgeons, Equipment & Supplies, and First Aid Supplies. Sources include

- surgical supply stores
- pharmacies

- hospitals
- home health care agencies
- medical supply catalogs

Where to Borrow

For short-term use, think about borrowing equipment from the following local groups:

- charity organizations
- faith-based groups, senior centers, leisure clubs
- home health care agencies
- National Easter Seal Society
- Red Cross
- Salvation Army
- Visiting Nurses Association

NOTE Never buy equipment from someone who calls you on the phone to sell you a product. Do not buy from a door-to-door salesperson. Do not buy from someone who calls you even before you know what equipment will be needed.

Checklist **General Supplies***

- ✓ antibacterial hand cleaner (kills germs)
- ✓ bacteriostatic ointment (stops the growth of germs)
- ✓ bandages, gauze pads, tape
- ✓ blankets (2 or 3)
- ✓ cotton balls and swabs
- ✓ toothbrush, toothpaste
- ✓ denture or dental care items
- ✓ kidney-shaped basin for oral care
- ✓ container for disposing of syringes (needles)
- ✓ disposable Chux underpad that keeps moisture out, for bed protection
- ✓ draw sheets for use in turning someone in bed
- ✓ finger towels and washcloths
- ✓ foam rubber pillows
- ✓ head pillows
- ✓ heating pad
- ✓ hydrogen peroxide
- ✓ ice bag
- ✓ lotion

- ✓ 4 bed sheets (at least)
- ✓ oral laxative
- ✓ poster with first aid procedures
- ✓ pressure pad and pump
- ✓ sterile disposable gloves
- ✓ rubbing alcohol
- ✓ seat belts (to prevent sliding down in a chair)
- ✓ shower cap
- ✓ soap for dry skin
- ✓ ear thermometer
- ✓ tissues
- ✓ disposable underpants
- ✓ incontinence briefs
- ✓ panty liners
- ✓ toilet paper tongs to take care of personal hygiene
- ✓ waterproof sheeting
- ✓ roll belt restraint
- ✓ gait/transfer belt
- ✓ Medic Alert® identification

*As needed.

How to Pay

If you need assistance in paying for medical equipment:

- Ask the doctor to write an order for a home evaluation (assessment), including an evaluation of needed equipment.

- Find out if the equipment is partly or completely covered by private health insurance with home care benefits.

- Check state retirement and union programs.

Medicare does not help pay for assistive devices, but does pay for durable medical equipment in some cases. To be covered, the equipment must be prescribed by a doctor and it must be medically necessary. It must be useful only to the sick or injured person and must be reusable. Medicare will pay for the rental of certain items for no more than 15 months. After that time you may buy the equipment from the supplier. If the person in your care has met the deductible, Medicare will pay 80% of the approved charges on the rental, purchase, and service of equipment that the doctor has ordered.

GETTING ORGANIZED

Keep supplies together that are used often and keep a list of supplies so you can easily replace them.

Be prepared for emergencies. Have on hand a flashlight, a battery-run radio, a battery-run clock, fresh batteries, extra blankets, candles with holders, matches, and a manual can opener.

Medical Equipment

You will need to have special equipment for different rooms in the house, as well as equipment to increase the person's ability to get around.

Equipment for the Bedroom

The equipment you need to have depends on the person's medical condition. This equipment might include some of the items listed below.

- **hospital bed**—allows positioning (adjusting) that is not possible in a regular bed and aids in resting and breathing more comfortably and getting in and out of bed more easily

- **alternating pressure mattress**—reduces pressure on skin tissue

- **egg-carton pad**—a foam mattress pad shaped like the bottom of an egg carton that reduces pressure and improves air circulation

- **portable commode chair**—for ease of toileting at the bedside

- **trapeze bar**—provides support and a secure hand-hold while changing positions

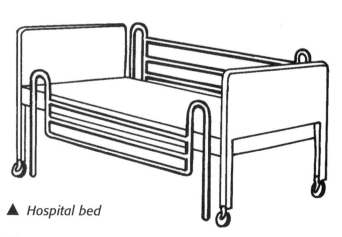

▲ *Hospital bed*

- **transfer board**—a smooth board for independent or assisted transfer from bed to wheelchair, toilet, or portable commode (📖 see p. 306)

- **hydraulic lift**—for use on a person who is difficult to move

- **over-the-bed table**—provides a surface for eating, reading, writing, and game playing (could be an adjustable ironing board)

- **mechanical or electric lift chair**—for help getting up from a chair

- **blanket support**—a wire support that keeps heavy bed linens off injured areas or the feet

- **urinal and bed pan**—for toileting in the bed

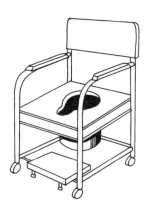

▲ *Portable commode chair*

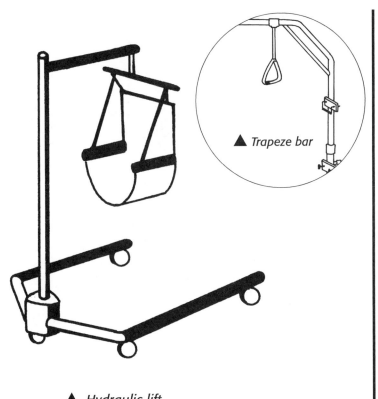

▲ *Trapeze bar*

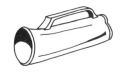

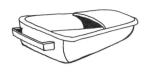

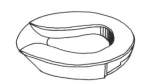

▲ *Urinal and bedpans*

▲ *Hydraulic lift*

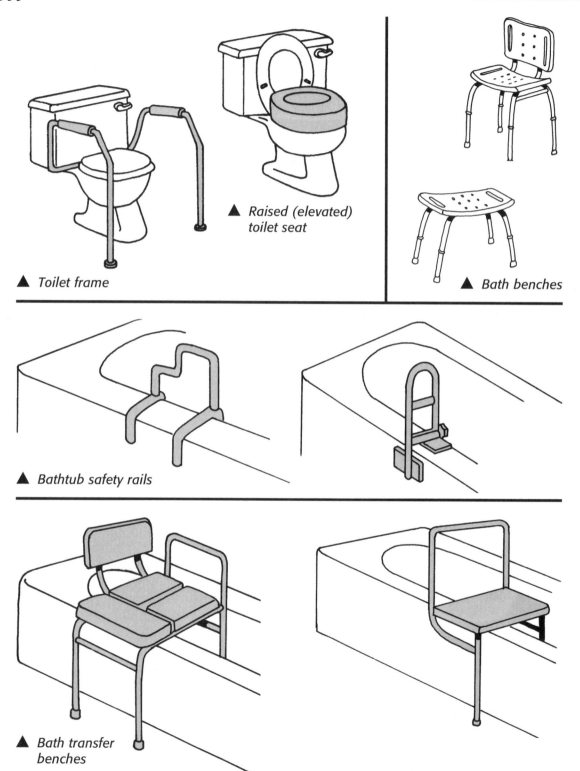

▲ Raised (elevated) toilet seat

▲ Toilet frame

▲ Bath benches

▲ Bathtub safety rails

▲ Bath transfer benches

Equipment for the Bathroom

The equipment you will need depends on the person's needs. You should consider providing the following:

- **raised (elevated) toilet seat**—used to assist a person who has difficulty getting up or down on a toilet (available in molded plastic and clamp-on models for different toilet bowl styles)

- **commode aid**—a device that acts as an elevated toilet seat when used with a splash guard, or as a commode when used with a pail

- **toilet frame**—a free-standing unit that fits over the toilet and provides supports on either side for ease in getting up and down

- **grab bars for tub and shower**—properly installed wall-mounted safety bars that hold a person's weight

- **safety mat and strips**—rough vinyl strips that stick to the bottom of the tub and shower to prevent slipping

- **hand-held shower hose**—a movable shower hose and head that allows the water to be directed to all parts of the body

- **bath bench**—aid for a person who has difficulty sitting down in or getting up from the bottom of the tub

- **bath transfer bench**—a bench that goes across the side of the tub and allows a person to get out of the tub easily

- **bathtub safety rails**—support for getting in and out of the tub

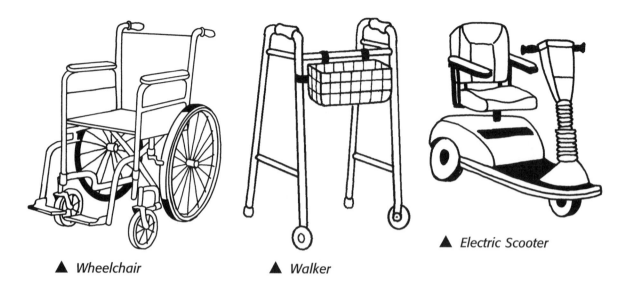

▲ Wheelchair   ▲ Walker   ▲ Electric Scooter

Mobility Aids

Mobility aids include devices that help a person move around without help. They also help the caregiver transfer the person in and out of bed and from bed to a chair.

They include—

▼ Canes

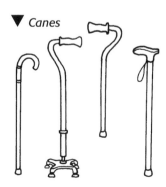

- a wheelchair with padding and removable arms

- a walker to help maintain balance and provide some support

- a 3- or 4-wheel electric scooter

- crutches when weight cannot be put on one leg or foot

- a cane to provide light weight-bearing support

- a transfer board (9″ x 24″) for moving someone in and out of bed (📖 see illustration p. 306)

- a gait/transfer belt (📖 see how to use on p. 303)

Wheelchair Requirements

Proper fit, as determined by a physical therapist.

- safety
- durability
- ease of repair
- attractive appearance

- comfort
- ease of handling
- cushions

Wheelchair Attachments for Stroke Survivors

- a brake lever extension on the handle
- elevated leg rests and removable footrests
- armrests that can be taken off

NOTE Some states have lemon laws that cover wheelchairs and other assistive devices. If you think there is something wrong with the equipment you have bought and you want to find out if it qualifies as a lemon, call the Attorney General's office in your state. They may be able to help you in getting a replacement or a refund.

Assistive Devices

For those with poor sight and hearing or other limitations, there are many aids to make life easier. Look into all the options and you will find that your job as caregiver becomes easier too.

Sight Aids

- prism glasses
- magnifying glasses
- prescription glasses
- Braille books and signs
- cassette players and books on tape
- telesensory devices that change printed letters into symbols that can be touched

Listening Aids

- hearing aids (order from an audiologist, or hearing therapist, who allows a free 30-day trial and is a registered dealer)
- sound systems that amplify (make louder)
- telephone amplifiers (for increased volume)
- devices for getting close-captioned TV programs

Tip — **HELP FOR SPECIAL EQUIPMENT**
Look into whether Medicaid or the Lion's Club in your state can pay for hearing aids.

Eating Aids

- spoons that swivel for those who have trouble with wrist movement

- foam that can be fit over utensils to increase the gripping surface so they can be lifted more easily

- plate guards or dishes with high sides that make it easier to scoop food onto a spoon

- rocker knives that can cut food with a rocking motion

- food-warming dishes for slow eaters

- mugs with two handles, a cover, a spout, and a suction base

▼ *Eating aids—mug, utensils with built-up handles, food guard, one-hand knife, swivel spoon*

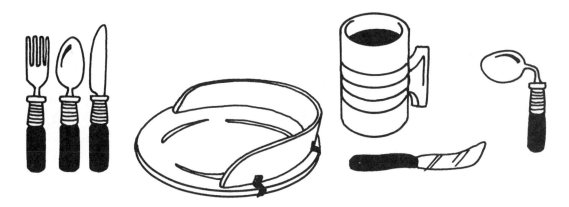

Dressing Aids

- button hooks that make buttoning clothes easy

- dressing sticks that make it possible to dress without bending

- long-handled shoehorns so a person doesn't have to bend over when putting on shoes

- sock aids that keep stockings open while they are being put on

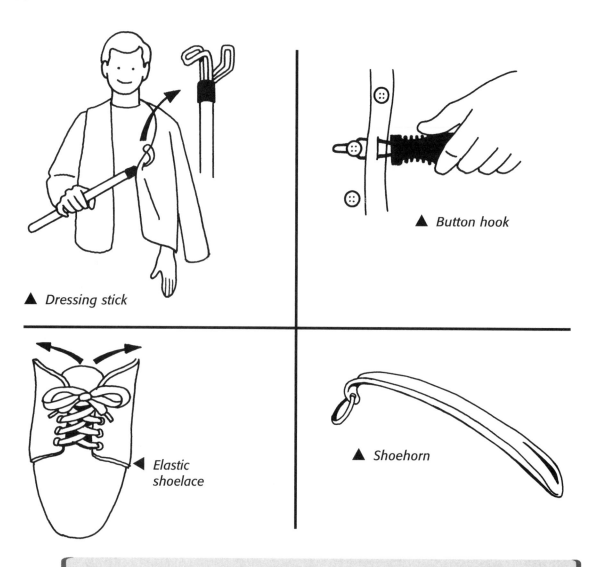

▲ Dressing stick

▲ Button hook

◀ Elastic shoelace

▲ Shoehorn

Tip

PUTTING ON SHOES
For people who have trouble tying laces, turn a lace-up shoe into a slip-on by replacing the cotton shoelaces with elastic ones.

Devices for Summoning Help

- touch-tone phones with speed dials

- medical security response systems
- beepers for the caregiver

Cooling Devices

Heat can be the enemy for many people. Learning how to "cool it!" in the summer months can be a problem. Fortunately, there are a number of cooling devices available to help the caregiver or survivor beat the heat:

- There are scarves and neck wraps that can be made cool by simply soaking in water.
- Cooling vests are another staple among cooling devices.
- There are devices for cooling wrists and ankles. One brand has arm and leg bands made of terrycloth into which you insert custom-size freezer packs.

Computer Equipment

There are countless hardware and software programs to make computers easier for people with disabilities to use. Alternative keyboards, puff switches for those who cannot use a mouse, screen readers, talking word processors, and voice recognition software are available today.

Homemade Aids and Gadgets

- wrist straps for canes—tape tied on a cane so it can be hung from the wrist while walking upstairs
- bicycle baskets—strapped to a walker to store necessities and leave the hands free
- an egg carton—to organize pills
- rubber safety mats—ideal for the tub, shower, or any slippery surface; also useful to make place on trays and tables for a nonslip surface

- key—put the end of the key that you hold into a large cork for ease of grip

- foot-operated door levers—made by attaching rope to a "stirrup" and tying it to the lever handle

- language tags—cardboard tags with words that can be used to express needs

- light-switch enlargements—made by putting a rubber pen cap over a light switch

- enlarged pull switches—made by putting a plastic ball over small switches

- clips for canes—spring clips or Velcro® placed on favorite chairs to keep a cane from falling

- bedside rails—wooden rails attached to the floor at right angles on swivel hinges

- pull rope—rope attached to the footboard of the bed to help someone change positions in bed

Equipment Cost-Comparison Chart *(Example)*

Item	Purchase Price	Rental Fee × Months Needed	Covered by Medicare Yes/No	Vendor
bath stool	$			
bed pan				
bed safety accessories				
cane				
commode				
crutches				
hospital bed				
mattress				
oxygen				
raised toilet seat				
special equipment				
trapeze				
walker				
wheelchair				
3- or 4-wheel scooter				
other				
Totals	$			

Specialized Hospital-Type Equipment

- **oxygen tanks**, for use when oxygen is needed as a medication

- **breathing tube (transtracheal oxygen therapy equipment)**, for use when oxygen is delivered into the lungs through a flexible tube that goes from the neck directly into the trachea (sometimes called the windpipe)

- **compressors and hand-held nebulizers (inhalers)**, which reduce medication to a form that can be inhaled

- **suction catheters**, which clear mucus and secretions from the back of the throat when someone cannot swallow

- **home infusion equipment**, or IV (intravenous) therapy, which delivers antibiotics, blood products, chemotherapy, hydration (water), pain management, parenteral (IV) nutrition, and specialty medications

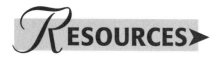
RESOURCES

AbilityHub
www.abilityhub.com
Assistive technology for people who have difficulty operating a computer.

ABLEDATA
8630 Fenton Street, Suite 930
Silver Spring, MD 20910-3319
(800) 227-0216; (301) 608-8998; Fax (301) 608-8958
www.abledata.com
Stores information on thousands of assistive devices for home health care, from eating utensils to wheelchairs. Provides prices, names, and addresses of suppliers.

Adaptive Environments Center Inc.
374 Congress Street, Suite 301
Boston, MA 02210
(617) 695-1225 (v/tty); Fax (617) 482-8099
www.adaptiveenvironments.org
E-mail: info@adaptiveenvironments.org

Alliance for Technology Access
www.ataccess.org
A network of community-based resource centers, developers, vendors, and associates dedicated to providing information and support services to children and adults with disabilities, and increasing their use of standard, assistive, and information technologies. You can order their book Computer Resources for People with Disabilities *online.*

American Occupational Therapy Association (AOTA)
4720 Montgomery Lane
P.O. Box 31220
Bethesda, MD 20824-1220
(301) 652-2682; Fax (301) 652-7711
www.aota.org
Provides consumer publications.

Apple Computer Accessibility
www.apple.com/accessibility
Committed to helping people with disabilities to access their computers.

AT&T Special Needs Center
Tel: (800) 872-3883 (TTY)
Provides free directory assistance (with an application) and operator's help dialing for those who are vision impaired and disabled.

Briggs
(800) 247-2343

Independent Living Research Utilization at TIRR
2323 S. Shepherd, Suite 1000
Houston, TX 77019
(800) 949-4232l; (713) 520-0232
www.ilru.org
E-mail: ilru@ilru.org

Lighthouse International
111 East 59th Street
New York, NY 10022-1202
(800) 829-0500; (212) 821-9200
www.lighthouse.org
E-mail: info@lighthouse.org
Provides free information on eye-related diseases and can refer individuals to resources in your community. Free catalog on low-vision aides. Includes link to Vision Connection, an interactive resource for latest information on vision; features "Help Near You" function, to find resources in your area.

Medic Alert®
(800) 432-5378
Offers critically important medical facts about the emblem wearer's condition to emergency personnel 24 hours a day.

Microsoft Accessibility Technology for Everyone
www.microsoft.com/enable
A Web site of products, training, and free resources to make technology accessible to everyone.

National Rehabilitation Information Center for Independence
4200 Forbes Boulevard, Suite 202
Lanham, MD 20706
(800) 346-2742
www.naric.com
E-mail: naricinfo@heitechservices.com
A database of research information about assistive technology and rehabilitation. One-stop shopping for referrals, information, and equipment sources. Fees for some services.

NCM Aftertherapy Catalog
(800) 235-7054

Radio Shack
Carries a variety of alerting devices in stores nationwide.
Check your phonebook for store near you.

Sammons-Preston
Bowling Brook, IL
(800) 323-5547

Sears Home Health Care Catalogue
(800) 326-1750 for customer service
To place an order or find a Sears store near you.

Self-Help for Hard of Hearing People (SHHH)
7910 Woodmont Avenue, Suite 1200
Bethesda, MD 20814
(301) 657-2248; (301) 657-2249 (TTY)
Offers information on coping with hearing loss and on hearing aids.

SpeciaLiving Magazine
www.specialiving.com
Online info and store for accessible housing, special products, such as ramps, bathing systems, urinary devices, lifts.

University of Florida—Project Link
P.O. Box 100164
Gainesville, FL 32610-0164
(877) 770-7303
www.phhp.ufl.edu/ot/projectlink
A nationwide information service, Project Link mails catalogs and brochures from different companies that manufacture assistive devices.

World Institute on Disability
510 16th Street, Suite 100
Oakland, CA 94612
(510) 763-4100; TTY: (510) 208-9496;
Fax: (510) 763-4109
www.wid.org
E-mail: wid@wid.org

For **medical alarms**, consult the phone book or contact your local hospital's long-term-care or senior services division.

If you don't have access to the Internet, ask your local library to help you locate a Web site.

Part Two: Day by Day

Chapter

Setting Up a Plan of Care

Setting Up a Plan of Care

$\mathcal{A}$ plan of care is a daily record of the care and treatment a person needs on a daily basis. The plan helps you and anyone who assists you with caregiving tasks.

A plan of care helps caregivers manage the day-to-day activities of the person in their care—medications, appointments, exercise, etc. This type of written record is also very helpful when respite (relief) care is used.

The plan of care includes the following information:

- diagnosis

- medications

- physical limitations of the care receiver

- a list of equipment needed

- diet

- detailed care instructions and comments

- services the home health care agency will provide, if using such on agency.

This information is presented in a certain order so that the process of care is repeated over and over again until it becomes routine. When the plan is kept up to date, it provides a clear record of events that is helpful in solving problems and avoiding them. With a plan you don't have to rely on your memory. It also allows another person to take over respite care or take your place entirely without too much trouble.

Some of the things you may have to watch and record are

- skin color, warmth, and tone (dryness, firmness, etc.)

- *pressure areas where bedsores can develop (See Activities of Daily Living, p. 187)*
- *breathing, temperature, pulse, and blood pressure*
- *circulation (dark red or blue spots on the legs or feet)*
- *finger and toenails (any unusual conditions)*
- *mobility (ability to move around)*
- *puffiness around the eyes and cheeks, swelling of the hands and ankles*
- *appetite*
- *body posture (relaxed, twisted, or stiff)*
- *bowel and bladder function (unusual changes)*

Recording the Plan of Care

To record the plan of care, use a loose-leaf notebook. Put the doctor's instructions on the inside front cover (always keep the originals). Include in the notebook the types of forms that appear in the following pages in this chapter. These pages should be three-hole punched.

After using your plan of care for one week, adjust as needed and keep doing so as the person's needs change. Always do what works for you and the person being cared for. Use notes, pictures, or anything else to describe your duties. Also, use black ink, not pencil, to keep a permanent record.

Daily Activities Record (Sample Form) Day/Date: _____

Morning _____

_____

Afternoon _____

_____

Naps: Time _____ Place _____

Evening _____

_____

Activities	Yes	No	Where/How/When
Walk	☐	☐	_____
TV	☐	☐	_____
Reading	☐	☐	_____
Visitors	☐	☐	_____
Calls to Friends/Relatives	☐	☐	_____
Other _____			_____

Bedtime Routine	Yes	No	Where/How
Incontinence Pad/Brief	☐	☐	_____
Medication	☐	☐	_____
Special Pillow/Blanket	☐	☐	_____
Music/Radio/TV	☐	☐	_____
Nightlight	☐	☐	_____
Restraints, Calming Techniques	☐	☐	_____
Urinal/Bedpan	☐	☐	_____
Gates at Doors/on Stairs	☐	☐	_____
Oral/Denture Care	☐	☐	_____
Foot Care	☐	☐	_____

Braces ☐   Fungus ☐   Massage ☐   Ingrown Nails ☐   Nail Care ☐

Meals

Help Needed with Meals _____

Meal Times _____

Special Diet _____

Foods to Avoid _____

Special Utensils _____

Snacks _____

Favorite Foods _____

Location of Meals _____

Daily Care Record (Sample Form)   Day/Date: _____

Daily Activities/Limitations:

Walks Alone _____ Stands Alone _____

Bed Position _____

Equipment Used: Walker ❑   Cane ❑   Wheelchair ❑   Brace ❑

How long _____

ROM/Exercises: Upper Body ❑   Lower Body ❑   Goes Outside ❑

Meals: Special Diet   ❑

Breakfast _____

Lunch _____

Dinner _____

Snack _____

Fluids _____

Treatments

Catheter _____

Oxygen _____

Equipment _____

Physical Therapy _____

Special Precautions _____

Resuscitate ❑   Do Not Resuscitate ❑

Personal Care

Bath: ❑ Bed   ❑ Chair

Shower: ❑ Tub   ❑ Bench

Care of Genitals: _____

Nail Care: ❑ Toes   ❑ Fingers

Oral Care: ❑ Brush Teeth   ❑ Floss Teeth   ❑ Dentures

Hair Care: ❑ Shave   ❑ Bed Shampoo   ❑ Bath/Shampoo

Skin Care: ❑ Lotion Upper Body   ❑ Lotion Lower Body   ❑ Powdered

Massage: ❑ Head and Shoulder   ❑ Leg and Foot   ❑ Back

Bowel Movements _____ Voiding _____ Quantity _____

Temperature _____ Blood Pressure _____ Respiration _____

Comments/Attitudes/Conditions _____

_____

Visitors _____

_____

Activities Schedule for Backup Caregiver (Sample Form)

Personal Needs	Yes	No	Where to Find
Cane	☐	☐	_____
Dentures	☐	☐	_____
Glasses	☐	☐	_____
Hearing aid	☐	☐	_____
Walker	☐	☐	_____
Other mobility device	☐	☐	_____

Morning Routine

Breakfast _____ Where Eaten _____

Amount of Help Needed _____

Special Utensils Needed _____

Medications with Meals ☐ _____ Nap ☐ _____

Snack Foods _____ Time of Snack _____

Evening Routine

Dinner _____ Where Eaten _____

Evening Snack _____

Bedtime Routine

Help Needed Undressing ☐ _____ Shower or Bath Needed ☐ _____

Where Clothes Are Stored _____

Where Dentures Are Stored _____

Special Items Needed: _____

Incontinent Pad/Brief ☐ _____ Urinal ☐ _____ Restraints ☐ _____

Special Pillows ☐ _____ Music ☐ _____ Nightlight ☐ _____

Calming Techniques _____

Special Concerns or Equipment

Catheter ☐ _____ Oxygen ☐ _____

Special Precautions _____

Other _____

Resuscitate ☐   **Do Not Resuscitate** ☐

Be on the Alert for:

Gates on Stairs/Locks on Doors _____

Alarms _____

Other _____

Don't be surprised if: _____

Recording and Managing Medications

You must have a careful system for keeping track of medications:

- when medications should be given
- how they should be given
- when they were actually given

The following sample of a weekly medication schedule is a good model to follow. Be sure to fill in the times (A.M. and P.M.) when medications actually were given, and have each caregiver initial them.

Weekly Medication Schedule (Sample Form)

Medication	Date/Time/Initials						
Name, dose, frequency, with food, without food	Sat.	Sun.	Mon.	Tues.	Wed.	Thurs.	Fri.
Disease-Modifying Therapy	Date/Time/Initials						
Name of Drug	Sat.	Sun.	Mon.	Tues.	Wed.	Thurs.	Fri.
Example							
2 mg. Coumadin 1× daily am with food	8:30am	8:00am	9:00am	8:45am	9:00am	8:30am	7:45am
400 mg. folic acid 1× daily am	8:30am	8:00am	9:00am	8:45am	9:00am	8:30am	7:45am
Fruitlax 1 Tbsp. evening only	6pm	6pm	6:30pm	6:45pm	6:15pm	6:30pm	7:00pm
Visine	10am	10am		4pm			

As you finish your own schedule, be sure to record information from the label of each prescription, including the following:

- days of the week when each medicine must be taken
- number of times per day
- time of day
- whether the medicine is to be taken with or without food
- how much water should be taken with the medicine

Also make a note to yourself about—

- any warnings (for example, "Don't take this medicine with alcohol")
- possible side effects (dizziness, confusion, headache, etc.)

> **NOTE**
>
> **Labels may contain the following abbreviations:**
>
> **HS**—Hour of sleep (medication time)
> **BID**—give the medicine 2 times per day (approximately 8am and 8pm)
> **TID**—give the medicine 3 times per day (approximately 9am, 1pm, 6pm)
> **QID**—give the medicine 4 times per day (approximately 9am, 1pm, 5pm, 9pm)

Other Cautions

- Never crush drugs without talking to the doctor or pharmacist. If the person in your care has trouble swallowing medication, ask the doctor for another way to give it. (See *Using the Health Care Team Effectively,* p. 66.)

- If the person in your care is going to take the medicine without your help, ask the pharmacist to prepackage dosages or come up with a color code to use when taking several medications.

- Do not store medicine that will be taken internally (swallowed) in the same cabinet with those that will be used externally (lotions, salves, creams, etc.).

- Keep a magnifying glass near the medicine cabinet for reading small print.

- Store most medicine in a cool, dry place—usually not the bathroom.

- Remove the cotton from each bottle so that moisture is not drawn in.

- Flush all medicine not currently being used down the toilet.

- Ask the pharmacist for containers that are not childproof if the childproof ones are too hard to open.

BEING READY FOR AN EMERGENCY

Notify the local fire station and ambulance company that a person with disabilities lives at this address. They will have the information on hand and can respond quickly.

Emergency Information

Have this information posted near telephones or on the refrigerator, where it can be used by anyone in the household in case of emergency.

Personal Information (Person in Your Care)

Name _____ Date of Birth _____

Address _____

Phone _____

SS # _____ Supplemental Insurance # _____

Medicaid # _____ Medicare # _____

Current Medications: _____

_____

Exact Location of Do Not Resuscitate Order: _____

Emergency Numbers

Fire _____ Police _____

Ambulance _____ Hospital _____

Doctor _____

Drugstore _____ Open Till _____ Delivers _____

Family Caregiver Work Number _____

Alternate Caregiver _____

Home Health Care Agency _____

Medicare Toll Free Number _____

Insurance _____

Medical Equipment Company _____

Poison Control _____

Friend _____

_____

Neighbor _____ Relative _____

Clergy/Rabbi _____

Transport Number _____ Meals-on-Wheels _____

Shopping Assistance _____

_____

Directions for Driving to the House _____

_____

_____

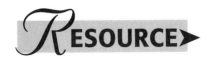

Elder Health Program
Peter Lamy Center on Drug Therapy and Aging
University of Maryland at Baltimore, School of Pharmacy
506 West Fayette Street, Room 106
Baltimore, MD 21201
(410) 706-2434; Fax (410) 706-1488
www.pharmacy.umaryland.edu/lamy
Provides free information about older people and medications.

If you don't have access to the Internet, ask your local library to help you locate a Web site.

How to Avoid Caregiver Burnout

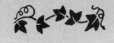

How to Avoid Caregiver Burnout

*P*roviding emotional support and physical care to a stroke survivor can be deeply satisfying, but it can be upsetting. Sometimes it is simply more than one person can handle. The strain of balancing a job, a family, more work in the home, and the care of someone may lead you to feel like a martyr or angry and guilty.

One of the biggest mistakes caregivers make is thinking that they can—and should—do everything by themselves. The best way to avoid burnout is to have the practical and emotional support of other people. Sharing concerns with others not only relieves stress, but also can give you a new slant on problems.

Negative Emotions That May Arise in You

The challenges of the caregiver role may sometimes make you feel bad about yourself. If you are a perfectionist, you'll never do it perfectly. If you're angry, you'll find plenty of excuses to be mad. If you have feelings of inadequacy, they'll definitely come up. Impatience, depression, hostility—if these emotions challenged you before, they're sure to arise in this situation.

Guilt Is Crippling

Opportunities for guilt can come up often in caregiving. Even if you are doing it perfectly, you can easily convince yourself that you're not doing enough. To combat this tendency, *at least once a day, every day*, remind yourself:

• about how you are helping your survivor

- when you don't do things perfectly, you are doing them with love

- you have grown in skill and compassion

Depression Is Dangerous

Just as depression endangers your survivor's recovery, it also endangers your health and well-being. Depression increases your risk in every major disease category, particularly cardiovascular disease.

Symptoms of Depression

Here again are the symptoms:

- persistent sad, anxious or "empty" mood

- feelings of hopelessness, pessimism

- feelings of guilt, worthlessness, helplessness

- loss of interest or pleasure in hobbies and activities that were once enjoyed, including sex

- decreased energy, fatigue, being "slowed down"

- difficulty concentrating, remembering, making decisions

- insomnia, early-morning awakening, or oversleeping

- appetite and/or weight changes

- thoughts of death or suicide, or suicidal attempts

- restlessness, irritability

If you have five or more of these symptoms for longer than two weeks, depression may be the cause. Talk to a physician, psychiatrist, or psychologist about treatment options. The most effective treatment combines medication with talking therapy.

> ***Tip***   Caring for your survivor can eat up all your time, if you let it.

- Claim time for yourself and make sure you use it; otherwise, you will burn out and your survivor will suffer.

- Make and keep doctor's appointments for yourself; otherwise, when you get sick, your survivor will suffer.

- Join a stroke or caregiver support group; otherwise, you and your survivor will suffer isolation.

- Take advantage of respite care opportunities, otherwise, when you break down your survivor will suffer.

Anger

It is easy to feel victimized in this situation; you are caught up in someone else's illness. The natural response is anger. Unfortunately, that is not a helpful response. Unleashing anger on the person in your care never helps.

On the other hand, it is not good for you to stuff those feelings. There are definite consequences to your health and well-being. Try these outlets:

- Caregiver support groups provide a place where you can vent feelings. Everyone there understands; no one will make you feel guilty. Members will often offer effective, real-world solutions. Scientific evidence indicates caregivers who participate in support groups are better able to deal with the situation.

- Make an appointment with a therapist or family counselor or clergyperson. If possible, make two appointments: one for you alone and one for you and your survivor.

- Keep a journal of your feelings.

- Remember, survivors who have lost control may try to regain it by controlling what they can, which may be their caregivers.

- Separate the person from the condition. The stroke, not the person in your care, is responsible for the difficulties and challenges that you both are facing. Don't blame the survivor for the situation you are in. *Remember, stroke changes behavior and personality.*

- Set and enforce limits on how many non-essential needs you will fill per hour, such as pouring water or changing channels. Non-emergency care does not have to be handled immediately.

Tip

Sometimes it is necessary to tell the survivor how you are feeling, but it is important not to accuse him personally. Saying "You make me feel angry" may worsen the situation. Instead say, "Just as I am trying to understand what you are going through, please try to understand what I am going through with you."

Emotional Burdens

You may think you are the only one to face these problems, but you are not alone. Every caregiver faces—

- the need to hide his or her grief

- fear of the future

- worries about money

- having less ability to solve problems

Dependency and Isolation

Fears of dependency and loneliness, or isolation, are common in families of those who are ill. The survivor can become more and more dependent on the one who is providing care. At the same time, the caregiver needs others for respite and support. Many caregivers are ashamed about needing help, so they don't ask for it. Those caregivers who are able to develop personal and social support have a greater sense of well-being.

NOTE Men who are caregivers face special problems. Often they are not used to doing daily chores around the house. They also lose the emotional support of the spouse who is ill and must now be her support. It is especially important for men to seek out a support system.

Knowing When to Seek Help

"**Why doesn't anyone ask how I am doing?**" It is easy to feel invisible, as if no one can see you. Everyone's attention is on the stroke survivor, and they don't seem to understand what the caregiver is going through. Many caregivers say that nobody even asks how they're doing. Mental health experts say it's not wise to let feelings of neglect build up. Caregivers need to speak up and tell other people what they need and how they feel.

Support groups, religious or spiritual advisors, or mental health counselors can teach you new and positive ways to express your own need for help.

Seek out professional help when you:

- are using more alcohol than usual to relax

- are using too many prescription medications

- have physical symptoms such as skin rashes, backaches, or a cold or flu that won't go away

- are unable to think clearly or focus

- feel tired and don't want to do anything

- feel keyed up and on edge

- feel sad all the time

- feel intense fear and anxiety

- feel worthless and guilty

- are depressed for two weeks or more

- are having thoughts of suicide

- have become or are thinking about becoming physically violent toward the person you are caring for

When Hostility Builds to the Breaking Point

Anger is a common emotion for caregivers and for the person being cared for. The situation feels—and is—unfair. Both may say hurtful words during a difficult task. Someone may slam a door during a disagreement. Shouting sometimes replaces conversation. Anger and frustration must be addressed and healthy outlets found as a way to let off steam. If they are not, angry situations can become physically or emotionally abusive.

You can control your emotions by letting go of anger and frustration in a safe way.

- Take a walk to cool down.

- Write your thoughts in a journal.

- Go to a private corner and take out your anger on a big pillow.

Checklist **Dealing with Physical and Emotional Burdens**

✓ Do not allow the person in your care to take unfair advantage of you by being overly demanding.

✓ Live one day at a time.

✓ List priorities, decide what to leave undone, and think of ways to make the work easier.

✓ When doing a long, boring care task, use the time to relax or listen to music.

✓ Find time for regular exercise to increase your energy (even if you only stretch in place).

✓ Focus on getting relaxing sleep rather than more sleep.

✓ Take several short rests in order to get enough sleep.

✓ Set aside time for prayer or reflection.

✓ Practice deep breathing and learn to meditate to empty your mind of all troubles.

✓ Allow your self-esteem to rise because you have discovered hidden skills and talents.

✓ Realize your own limitations and accept them.

✓ Make sure your goals are realistic—you may be unable to do everything you could do before.

✓ Keep your eating habits balanced—do not fall into a toast-and-tea habit.

✓ Take time for yourself.

✓ Treat yourself to a massage.

✓ Keep up with outside friends and activities.

✓ Spread the word that you would welcome some help, and allow friends to help with respite care.

✓ Delegate (assign) jobs to others. Keep a list of tasks you need to have done and assign specific ones when people offer to help.

✓ Share your concerns with a friend.

✓ Join a support group, or start one (to share ideas and resources).

✓ Use respite care when needed.

✓ Express yourself openly and honestly with people you feel should be doing more to help.

✓ When you visit your own doctor, be sure to explain your caregiving responsibilities, not just your symptoms.

✓ Allow yourself to feel your emotions without guilt. They are natural and very human.

✓ Unload your anger and frustration by writing it down.

✓ Allow yourself to cry and sob.

✓ Know that you are providing a very important service to the person in your care.

Where to Find Professional Help or Support Groups

- the community pages of the phone directory
- the local county medical society, which can provide a list of counselors, psychologists, and psychiatrists
- religious service agencies
- community health clinics
- religious and spiritual advisors
- United Way's "First Call for Help"
- a hospital's social service department
- a newspaper calendar listing of support group meetings
- parish nurses
- Area Agency on Aging

Ask for help from a counselor who is familiar with the needs of caregivers.

Self-Care for Caregivers

If you don't take care of yourself, then you won't finish the caregiving race, and your survivor will suffer. Part of your responsibility to the person in your care is to take care of yourself.

Tip Here's a thought to keep in mind: In the safety talk before every flight, the stewardess tells parents to put the oxygen mask on themselves first and then the child. Why? Because if the parent passes out, the child's safety is at risk.

Exercise

Even moderate exercise is beneficial because it breaks the cycle of being sedentary. And being sedentary is a risk factor for all major diseases.

Walking is easy, and if you can't walk for 30–40 minutes at a stretch, several 5–10 minute periods are enough. Exercise improves mood and physique and can be an opportunity to socialize. Find a way to make it part of your day.

Tip If you can't join a gym, investigate the YMCA. Some larger churches often have low- or no-cost exercise classes.

Eat Right

Nutrition is critical to your well-being. Learn to read labels and avoid foods with high fat content. Monitor your portion size; for example, a proper serving of meat is about the size of a deck of playing cards.

Your survivor will almost certainly be given a dietary prescription. In cooking heart-healthy for him, you will benefit yourself and the rest of your family. (See **Diet, Nutrition, and Exercise,** p. 262.)

Tip Calorie-dense foods pack a lot of calories in a small package—think chocolate. For example, 8 oz of broccoli is 65 calories; 8 oz of chocolate chip cookies is 1,070 calories. Fresh fruits and vegetables will typically have many fewer calories than processed foods. Canned fruit often has added sugar; canned vegetables generally have added salt.

> **Tip** Most people need to eat more fruit—9 servings a day. To help you meet that goal, keep a bowl of apples, oranges, pears, bananas, and seasonal fruits on a kitchen counter and nibble on the fruit throughout the day.

> **Tip** For reliable and easy-to-understand information on nutrition; changing your diet; easy-to-follow eating plans; and quick, tasty, and healthy recipes, go to www.American Heart.org. It is a free, one-stop shop for heart-healthy nutrition.

Take Care of the Caregiver

Many caregivers neglect their own physical health. They ignore what is ailing them and don't take steps to avoid getting sick, such as exercising, eating a proper diet, and getting regular medical examinations.

Many caregivers do not get enough sleep at night. If sleep is regularly broken up because the survivor needs help during the night, talk about the problems with a healthcare professional.

Your survivor needs a healthy caregiver. Both partners need uninterrupted sleep.

Meditation

Your journey as a caregiver will be more satisfying and less stressful if you take up a practice of daily meditation.

Think of meditation as sitting still doing nothing. Here are seven easy steps:

1. Sit so your back is straight, either on a chair or a big, firm pillow.

2. As you inhale, tense your whole body—arms, legs, buttocks, fists, scrunch your face.

3. Hold 2–3 seconds.

4. Exhale and relax (repeat twice).

5. Take a deep breath, let your belly expand.

6. Exhale and relax (repeat twice).

7. Breathe normally and observe your thoughts for five minutes.

Tip Most people fail at meditation because they think meditation means clearing your mind of thoughts. Instead of emptying your mind of thoughts, observe them. There are no "right" thoughts to think. Don't focus on any of your thoughts and don't fight with any of them. An easy way to do that is to label each one as it bubbles up—sad thought, happy thought, angry thought, depressed thought, to-do list thought—and let it go and then label the next one that appears.

Tip A kitchen timer will alert you to five minutes.

It is not important how long you sit with your eyes closed and observe your thoughts—5 minutes will do, especially to start. What makes meditation effective at reducing stress is the *practice* of meditation, doing it every day. You can do it before your survivor wakes up or after she goes to bed or is taking a nap. It's only 5 or 10 minutes, but the cumulative effect over just a few weeks is noticeable. (For more on meditation, visit www.mycalmspace.com.)

Plan for the Long Term: Winning the Caregiving Race

Most people jump into caregiving as if it were a sprint. They think they can and must do everything themselves.

You may be able to do that for a few weeks or even months, but the average caregiver spends more than four years in that role—no one can sprint for that long.

Instead of a sprint, treat caregiving as a marathon—for which you have not trained—and pace yourself accordingly from the start. Find effective ways to share or get help from others.

Tip If you find yourself in an angry conversation with your survivor *in your head*, get it out in the open.

- Find a counselor or therapist to talk to.

- Talk to a neutral third party, even if it's by phone or e-mail.

- Tap into a local or online support group.

- Keep a journal.

Respite Time

Every caregiver needs respite time if she is to last. It may be hard to think of yourself and your needs at this time, but if you don't, your life will be consumed by your duties and you will burn out. Respite (a temporary break from responsibility) is not a luxury, it is a necessity.

Your survivor's level of disability determines whether he or she can be left alone and for how long. Care options include—

- asking a family member or friend to stay with your survivor for an hour or two

- taking him or her to adult daycare (if ambulatory)

- employing a professional sitter or health care aide for a few hours a week or month

- hiring a college student (if skilled care is not needed) to stay with your survivor

- enrolling your survivor in a stroke support group

Check with your local Area Agency on Aging for respite-care programs in your area. Larger churches often have outreach programs that include respite care.

However you are able to arrange for your survivor's care—and it will take some effort on your part, it won't happen by itself—commit to taking some time at least once a week to do something for yourself.

NOTE To make this happen you will have to defend this time because other things will demand to be made a priority. If you do not defend your respite time, you will not get it or the renewal it generates. Remember, caregiving is a marathon, not a sprint—respite time helps you finish the race.

Respite Zone

A respite zone is an area within your home set aside just for you, the caregiver. The idea is that this is your space. It can be your bedroom, the spare room, an office, or even a bench outside in the garden or on a porch. This is a place for you to take a break while your survivor rests or is taken care of by someone else.

In creating your respite zone,

- Keep in mind what you want to do there. Reading? Painting? Writing? Gardening? Bubble bath?

- Identify the time you will use it—during nap time, when someone spells you? If you can only get a break at night after your survivor is in bed, gardening probably won't do.

- Identify free space in your home—porches are good candidates, a spare room is perfect, maybe a corner of your bedroom. A screen can give you privacy if you can't close the door.

- Modify the space according to your needs—a reading chair with a lamp or a stereo headset. Keep whatever is necessary for your respite activity.

Your respite zone should be your creation alone. The goal is to give you a place of your own where you can find enjoyment in your own home and life. If searching the Internet is fun for you, your zone will be different from someone who wants to take a bubble bath and listen to soft music. Creative projects such as painting, sewing, writing, baking, gardening, and photography are excellent ways to absorb your attention and take your mind off your responsibilities.

Your respite zone should be just for you. You need to feel secure that your things are safe and will not be disturbed or discarded. It is important for your survivor to understand that this space is yours.

 Tip It is not selfish to set aside space and time for yourself, because if you fail to give yourself space, time, and the opportunity to be with your own thoughts, your caregiving journey will be harder on you than it has to be.

Taking care of a debilitated (weakened) family member or friend who may not recover completely can be an all-consuming job. However, if you allow it to consume all of you because you do not demand some time and space for yourself, what will happen to your survivor when you collapse?

Respite care is not a luxury. It is necessary for your survivor's and your well-being.

Changes in Attitude Relieve Stress

Here are some suggestions to help reduce your stress level:

- Learn to say no. Good boundaries improve relationships.

- Control your attitude: Don't dwell on what you lack or what you can't change.

- Appreciate what you have and can do.

- Go on a TV diet. Find simple ways to have fun: Play a board game, organize family photos, listen to music you enjoy, read the biography of an inspiring person.

- Learn a time-management tool, like making a to-do list (specifically include items that you enjoy).

- Knowledge is empowering; get information about your survivor's condition.

- Limit coffee and caffeine.

- Find a support system and nurture it.

- Share your feelings with someone who wants to listen.

- Keep a gratitude journal—record three new things you are grateful for every day.

- Memorize an inspiring poem.

NOTE The #1 thing you can do to improve your situation is to acknowledge your role. A survey of family caregivers by the National Family Caregivers Association showed that spouse caregivers often refuse to accept that caregiving is a separate role to the role of spouse. The survey found that shifting this attitude—accepting that caregiving is a separate role—had a profound impact on their situation.

The job of long-term caregiving is too big for one person—no matter how much love the caregiver has for the survivor. Ask for and accept help from as many sources as you can find.

Outside Activities

Successful caregivers don't give up their own enjoyable activities. Many organizations have respite care programs to provide a break for caregivers. Other family members are often willing—even pleased—to spend time with the survivor. It may be possible to have respite care on a regular basis. Keep a list of the people you can ask for help once in a while.

If your friends want to know how they can help ease your burden, ask them to:

- telephone and be a good listener as you may voice strong feelings

- offer words of appreciation for your efforts

- share a meal

- help you find useful information about community resources

- show genuine interest

- stop by or send cards, letters, pictures, or humorous newspaper clippings

- share the workload

- help hire a relief caregiver

It helps to remember the saying, "Grant me the serenity to accept the things I cannot change, the courage to change the things I can, and the wisdom to know the difference."

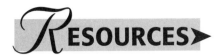

RESOURCES

Caregiver.com
www.caregiver.com
Maintains one of the most visited caregiver sites on the Internet. Publishes Today's Caregiver Magazine. *Provides links to many resources such as government and non-profit agencies.*

Caregiver Survival Resources
www.caregiver911.com
A comprehensive list linking caregiving information and services for general issues and specific chronic illnesses.

Center for Family Caregivers/Tad Publishing Co.
www.caregiving.com or www.familycaregivers.org
Develops and distributes educational materials on caregiving, including a newsletter. Caregiving informational kits are $5 each; please specify new, seasoned, and transitioning caregiver when requesting a kit.

Eldercare Locator
(800) 677-1116
www.eldercare.gov
Provides information about local support resources offering services to the elderly.

Lotsa Helping Hands
www.lotsahelpinghands.com
Provides a free-of-charge Web service that allows family, friends, neighbors, and colleagues to assist more easily with daily meals, rides, shopping, baby-sitting, and errands that may become a burden during times of medical crisis.

National Alliance for Caregiving
4720 Montgomery Lane, 5th Floor
Bethesda, MD 20184
www.caregiving.org
The Alliance is a non-profit coalition of national organizations focusing on issues of family caregiving.

National Family Caregivers Association
10400 Connecticut Avenue, Suite 500
Kensington, MD 20895
(800) 896-3650
info@thefamilycaregiver.org
www.thefamilycaregiver.org
Free member benefits include Take Care!, *a quarterly newsletter;* The Resourceful Caregiver, *a useful guide to resources; a support hotline and online chat room.*

Today's Caregiver Magazine
6365 Taft Street, Suite 3003
Hollywood, FL 33024
(800) 829-2734
www.caregiver.com/magazine
Bimonthly magazine dedicated to caregivers.

Well Spouse Association
63 West Main Street, Suite H
Freehold, NJ 07728
(800) 838-0879
info@wellspouse.org
www.wellspouse.org
Publishes Mainstay, *a bimonthly newsletter and provides networking/local support groups.*

Check with your local church or health facility to see if they sponsor **Share the Care** teams.

Publications

Care for the Family Caregiver: A Place to Start, a report prepared by HIP Health Plan of New York and National Alliance for Caregiving. Available at www.caregiving.org

The Emotional Survival Guide for Caregivers: Looking After Yourself and Your Family While Helping an Aging Parent by Barry J. Jacobs, PsyD. The Guilford Press.

Helping Yourself Help Others: A Book for Caregivers, by Rosalynn Carter, with Susan Golant. Random House/ Time Books, 1995.
(800) 733-3000
Plenty of basic information for caregivers.

Love, Honor and Value: A Family Caregiver Speaks Out about the Choices and Challenges of Caregiving, by Suzanne Geffen Mintz.

Mainstay: For the Well Spouse of the Chronically Ill by Maggie Strong.

Positive Caregiver Attitudes by James Sherman, PhD.

If you don't have home access to the Internet, ask your local library to help you locate any Web site.

For stroke-specific and additional Caregiver Organizations see p. 327.

Activities of Daily Living

Activities of Daily Living

One-Handed Tips

Stroke often leaves survivors with weakness or slight paralysis on one side of the body (hemiparesis) or complete paralysis of one side (hemiplegia). Often, function of the affected side can be brought back to some degree through rehab.

> **NOTE** A promising development in rehab specifically addresses this problem. Called *"constraint-induced therapy,"* it works by restraining the able side and requiring the affected side to do a movement or task for a substantial number of repetitions over an extended period of time. This therapy has proven effective in returning function to affected limbs even years after a stroke.

Helping your survivor adapt to being one-handed may challenge you, but much of his independence depends on it. The more things he can do by himself, the better for everyone. The tips that follow are some adaptations to everyday tasks that will help. They were adapted from the American Stroke Association booklet *Living with Disability After Stroke: Our Guide of Practical Tips for Daily Living.* It is available (with many more tips) for free by calling 1-888-4-STROKE (478-7653) or going online to www.AmericanStroke.org.

Grooming Tips

Teeth

Applying Toothpaste

- Instead of applying toothpaste to a toothbrush, it may be easier to squeeze it directly on the tongue.

- Balance the toothbrush in the overflow hole of the sink and squeeze toothpaste onto the bristles.

- Use an electric toothbrush. Most are flat on one side and allow the bristles to point up. Place your affected hand on the handle to stabilize it while applying toothpaste.

- Flip-top lids and pump-style toothpaste containers may be easier to use.

Flossing

- Use disposable flossing toothpicks. Available in the dental section of grocery or drug stores, they look like a miniature coping saw (a saw with a U-shaped frame) with a plastic handle. The "blade" is a piece of dental floss.

 Tip Brushing teeth or dentures twice a day may make food taste better.

Shaving

Men

- Use an electric razor.

- If using a standard razor, use a disposable so there is no need to change blades.

- Shaving cream can be squeezed on the side of the sink, or onto the back of the affected hand and applied with the other hand.

Women

- To shave legs, use an electric razor and lie on the bed so free movement is possible.

- To shave under the affected arm, rig a noose strap (a strap with a loop, tied with a knot that permits loosening and tightening of the loop) over the shower rod and place the affected arm in it. The strap can then be used as a pulley to lift the arm for shaving.

 Tip A roll-on hair remover may be easier than shaving.

Bathing

General Tips

- Showers are safer than tubs because there is less chance of falling when getting in and out.

- If you must use a tub, use a special seat from a medical equipment store that can be put on the tub rim.

- Bath benches can make showering easier. (See *Equipment and Supplies,* p. 129.)

- Have grab bars installed in the shower. Use non-skid tape or a rubber bath mat on the bottom of the tub or shower.

One-Handed Tips

- Adapt the shower with a hand-held showerhead with hose. This makes it easier to wash underarms and private areas.

- Instead of a loose bar of soap, put soap in a nylon stocking and attach it to a grab bar.

- Use a long-handled sponge or brush to wash back, legs, and feet.

- Pump bottles of liquid soap may work better for getting soap on a washcloth.

- Sew two washcloths together on three sides to make a pocket for holding a bar of soap.

- To wring out a washcloth press it against the side of the sink with the good hand; or drape it over the faucet and twist it.

- To wash the unaffected arm while sitting on a bath bench, hold the washcloth between the knees and move your arm back and forth over it.

- Instead of trying to rub dry the whole body after bathing, slip into a terry-cloth robe, along with a pair of slipper socks. Or, sew two large towels together and throw them around the shoulders.

- To apply deodorant under the affected arm, lean slightly forward, allowing the arm to dangle and then apply roll-on deodorant.

Dressing and Undressing Tips

 NOTE Getting up and getting dressed is important. It affects both mood and self-esteem. Insist that your survivor get out of his or her pajamas every day. Only sick people stay in their pajamas all day!

- When dressing, always put clothing on the affected side *first*. When undressing, always take clothes off the affected side *last*.

- Clothing that must be pulled over the head (undershirts, nightgowns, sweaters) may be difficult to manage.

- When getting dressed, lay out clothes in the order they will be put on. Those to be put on first go on top of the pile.

- Putting on clothes is easier when sitting than when lying down.

Putting on Panty Hose

- While seated, cross the affected leg over the unaffected leg. Gather up the stocking for the affected leg in the unaffected hand, all the way to the toe.

- Put the stocking over the toes and foot. Uncross the legs and pull the stocking to the knee.

- Gather the other stocking leg to the toes and put it over the toes of the unaffected leg and start pulling up the stocking.

- Stand up to pull panty hose completely up or lie on the bed and roll side to side.

- Buy a size larger than normal—they go on easier or buy thigh-high nylons that use an elastic band to hold them in place.

Shoes

- There are several products available for tying shoes. Investigate assistive-device catalogs.

- Have a shoe repair shop alter the shoes by installing Velcro closures.

- For help putting on socks, buy a sock stretcher through one of the assistive-device catalogs. Using a larger-size sock also helps.

- If using a brace, put the brace in the shoe first. Pick up the shoe by the toe and lay it down on the back of the brace. Step into the trough (long, narrow opening) of the brace and slide the foot forward into the shoe. Hold the tongue out of the way.

Belts

- Put the belt on the skirt, slacks, or dress before putting it on.

Putting on Pants

- Rather than trying to pull pants on holding the waist in weak fingers, thrust the affected hand deep into the side pocket and pull up the pants. This allows the arm to hold the weight of the pants rather than the fingers.

- Use the unaffected hand to put in the shirttails.

- To close the waist, put the affected thumb through the last belt loop then push against that to draw the waist closer together.

Eating

- A rocker knife makes it easier to cut food. Check out assistive-device catalogs for other one-handed eating utensils. (📖 See *Equipment and Supplies*, p. 141.)

- For hands with poor grip strength, a piece of sponge rubber over the handle of the eating utensil makes it easier to grasp.

- Use non-skid shelf paper to keep plates, bowls, and cups from sliding.

- If one side of the mouth lacks feeling, swallowing may be affected. Put small amounts of food in the unaffected side of the mouth. This will make swallowing easier and help prevent choking.

- Food may tend to become lodged in the affected side of the mouth. The survivor can check for trapped food with a mirror and remove it with tongue or fingers.

- When eating out, order food that is easy to eat and cut (for example, chopped steak or fish fillets). Or request that the meat be cut into bite-size pieces in the kitchen.

- Try chopsticks; they only require one hand.

Personal Hygiene

As a caregiver, you may find that some of your time each day will be devoted to assisting the person in your care with personal hygiene. This includes bathing, shampooing, oral or mouth care, shaving, and foot care.

The Bed Bath

Bed baths are needed by people who are confined to bed. Baths clean, stimulate, and increase blood flow (circulation) in the skin. However, they can also dry the skin and in some instances cause chapping. Thus, you must decide how often a bed bath is needed. Your decision must be based on the situation of the person in your care. For example, if urinary incontinence (leakage), bowel problems, and heavy perspiration are present, a daily bath may be in order. If not, bathing 2 to 3 times a week might be enough. At bath time, inspect the whole body for pressure sores, swelling, rashes, moles, and other unusual conditions. If baths are given often and the skin is dry, use soap and water one time and lotion and water the next. Cornstarch and powder can cause skin problems in some people. Ask the nurse on your health care team for advice.

Tip

SKIN CARE
It is easier to prevent chapping than to heal it, so apply lotion often.

To avoid spreading germs, always wash your own hands before and after giving a bath. At each step, tell the person what you are about to do and ask for his help if he is able. (📖 See *One-Handed Tips*, p. 188)

1. Make sure the room is a comfortable temperature and not too warm.

2. Gather supplies—disposable gloves, mild soap, washcloth, washbasin, lotion, comb, electric razor, shampoo—and clean clothes.

3. Use good body mechanics (position)—keep your feet separated, stand firmly, bend your knees, and keep your back in a neutral position. (See *Body Mechanics—Positioning, Moving, and Transfers*, p. 290.)

4. Offer the bedpan or urinal.

5. If you have a hospital bed, raise the bed to its highest level and bring the head of the bed to an upright position.

6. Help with oral hygiene—brushing the teeth or cleansing the mouth. (See p. 204.)

7. Test the temperature of the water in the basin with your hand.

8. Remove the person's clothes, the blanket, and the top sheet. Cover the person with a towel or light blanket. Keep all of the body covered during the bed bath, uncovering only one area at a time while washing it.

9. Now have the person lie almost flat.

10. Use one washcloth for soap, one for rinsing, and a dry towel. Have the washcloth very damp, but not dripping.

11. Very gently wash the face first; pat dry.

NOTE Always start washing at the cleanest part and work toward the dirtiest part.

12. Wash the front of the neck; pat dry.

13. Wash the chest, and for females under the breasts; pat dry.

14. Wash the stomach and upper thighs; pat dry.

15. Clean the navel with a little lotion on a cotton swab.

16. Wash upward from wrist to upper arm to increase circulation; pat dry.

17. Wash the hands and between the fingers; check the nails; pat dry.

18. Place a towel under the person's buttocks.

19. Flex (bend) the person's knees.

20. Wash the legs; pat dry.

21. Wash the feet and between the toes and dry well. Use lotion on dry feet. Do not put lotion between toes. This area must be kept dry and clean to prevent fungal infection.

22. Wash the pubic area. If possible, have the person wash his or her own genitals; if not, do it yourself. (Use PeriWash to prevent a buildup of germs.)

23. If a male is not circumcised, draw back the foreskin, rinse, dry, and bring the foreskin down over the head of the penis again. For the female, wash the genitals thoroughly by spreading the external folds. (This must be done at least daily.)

24. Pat the genitals dry.

25. Watch for unusual tenderness, swelling, or hardness in the testicles.

26. Change the bath water.

27. Roll the person away from you.

28. Tuck a towel under the person.

29. Wash the back from the neck to the buttocks.

30. Rinse; dry well.

31. Give a back rub with lotion to improve circulation.

32. Dress the person.

33. Change the bed linens.

34. Trim the toenails if they are long.

> **NOTE** A buildup of earwax may obstruct hearing. Have the ears checked and cleaned by a nurse or doctor twice a year. If the doctor approves, apply a little lotion to the outside of the ears to prevent drying and itching.

The Basin Bath

If the person in your care can be in a chair or wheelchair, you can give a sponge bath at the sink.

1. Make sure the room is warm.

2. Gather supplies—disposable gloves, mild soap, washcloth, washbasin, lotion, comb, electric razor, shampoo—and clean clothes.

3. Use good body mechanics (position)—keep your feet separated, stand firmly, bend your knees, and keep your back in neutral. (See *Body Mechanics—Positioning, Moving, and Transfers*, p. 290.)

4. Offer the urinal.

5. Wash the face first.

6. Wash the rest of the upper body.

7. If the person can stand, wash the genitals. If the person is too weak to stand, wash the lower part of the body in the bed.

The Tub Bath

If the person in your care has good mobility and is strong enough to get in and out of the tub, he or she may enjoy a tub bath. Be sure there are grab bars, a bath bench, and a rubber mat so the person doesn't slide. (It may be easier to sit at bench level rather than at the bottom of the tub.) Use the following steps:

1. Make sure the room is a comfortable temperature.

2. Gather supplies—disposable gloves for the caregiver, mild soap, washcloth, lotion, comb, electric razor, shampoo—and clean clothes.

3. Check the water temperature before the person gets in.

4. Guide the person into the tub. Have the person use the grab bars. (Don't let the person grab you and pull you down.)

5. Help the person wash.

6. Empty the tub and then help the person get out.

7. Guide the person to use the grab bars while getting out. OR you can have the person stand up and then sit on the bath bench. Swing first one leg, then the other leg, over the edge of the tub. Help him stand.

8. Put a towel on a chair or the toilet lid and have the person sit there to dry off.

9. Apply lotion to any skin that appears dry.

10. Help the person dress.

BATHING IN THE TUB
If a bath bench is not used, many people feel more secure if they turn on to their side and then get on their knees before rising from the tub. This is a very helpful way to get out of the tub if the person is unsteady.

The Shower

Before starting, be sure the shower floor is not slippery. Also make sure there are grab bars, a bath bench, and a rubber mat so the person doesn't slide. A removable shower head is also useful.

1. Make sure the room is a comfortable temperature.

2. Explain to the person what you are going to do.

3. Provide a shower stool in case he or she needs to sit.

4. Gather supplies—mild soap, washcloth, washbasin, comb, electric razor, shampoo—and clean clothes.

5. Turn on the cold water and then the hot to prevent burns. Test and adjust the water temperature before the person gets in. Use gentle water pressure.

6. First, spray and clean the less sensitive parts of the body such as the feet.

7. For safety, ask the person to hold the grab bar or to sit on the shower stool.

8. Move the water hose around the person rather than asking the person to move.

9. Assist in washing as needed.

10. Guide the person out of the shower and wrap with a towel. Turn the water off.

11. Apply lotion to skin that appears dry.

12. If necessary, have the person sit on a stool or on the toilet lid.

13. Assist in drying and dressing.

 NOTE Remove from the bathing area all electrical equipment that could get wet.

Nail Care

When providing nail care, you can watch for signs of irritation or infection. This is especially important in a person with diabetes, for whom a small infection can develop into something more serious. Fingernails and toenails can thicken with age, which will make them more difficult to trim.

1. Assemble supplies—soap, basin with water, towel, nailbrush, scissors, nail clippers, file, and lotion.

2. Wash your hands.

3. Wash the hands of the person in your care with soap and water and soak the hands in a basin of warm water for 5 minutes.

4. Gently scrub the nails with the brush to remove trapped dirt.

5. Dry the nails and gently push back the skin around the nails (the cuticle) with the towel.

6. To prevent ingrown nails, cut nails straight across.

7. File gently to smooth the edges.

8. Gently massage the person's hands and feet with lotion.

 If other members of the household are using the same equipment, clean the nail clippers with alcohol.

Shampooing the Hair

Keeping the hair and scalp clean improves blood flow to the scalp and keeps the hair healthy. Women especially may consider it a special treat to have their hair styled. Shampooing can be done anytime the person in your care is not overly tired. Before a bath may be the most convenient time. Adopt a system that is easiest for you and the person in your care.

SHAMPOOING

To make washing easy, dilute the shampoo in a bottle before pouring it on the hair.

Wet Shampoo

1. Assemble supplies—disposable gloves, comb and brush, shampoo/conditioner, several pitchers of warm water, large basin, washcloth, towels.

2. Have the person sit on a chair or commode.

3. Drape a large towel over the person's shoulders.

4. Gently comb out any knots.

5. Protect the person's ears with cotton.

6. Ask the person to cover his or her eyes with a washcloth and to lean over the sink.

7. Moisten the hair with a wet washcloth or with water poured from a pitcher.

8. Massage a small amount of diluted shampoo into the hair.

9. Remove the shampoo with clean water or a washcloth until the rinse water or cloth runs clear.

10. Use a leave-in conditioner if desired.

11. Towel the hair dry.

12. Remove the cotton from the ears.

13. Comb the hair gently.

14. If desired, use a hair dryer on the cool setting to dry hair, being very careful not to burn the scalp.

OR

1. Cut a round slit at the raised edge of a heavy rubber dish-draining mat so that the end can tuck under the person's neck and the water can drain down into the sink.

2. Seat the person at the kitchen sink with her back to the mat.

3. Place a towel on the person's shoulders and place the rubber dish-draining mat with the round cut against the neck and the smooth edge draining into the sink (beauty salon style).

4. Follow the procedure above, using the sink hose or a pitcher to wash and rinse the hair.

Dry Shampoo

1. Assemble supplies—disposable gloves for the caregiver, comb and brush, waterless shampoo, and towels.

2. Lather the head until all foam disappears.

3. Towel the hair dry and gently comb it.

> **NOTE** You can buy a waterless shampoo from the pharmacy or at a medical supply company.

Wet Shampoo in Bed

1. Assemble supplies—disposable gloves, comb and brush, shampoo/conditioner, several pitchers of warm water, a large basin, plastic sheet, washcloth, towels, and hair dryer.

2. If possible, raise the bed.

3. Help the person lie flat.

4. Protect the bedding with plastic under the head and shoulders.

5. Roll the edges of the plastic inward so the water will run down into a basin placed on a chair next to the head of the bed.

6. Drape a towel over the person's shoulders.

7. Protect the person's ears with cotton.

8. Cover the person's eyes with a washcloth.

9. Moisten the hair with a wet washcloth.

10. Massage a small amount of diluted shampoo into the hair.

11. Remove the shampoo with a wet washcloth until the water runs clear when the cloth is wrung out.

12. Use leave-in conditioner if desired.

13. Towel the hair dry.

14. Remove the cotton from the ears.

15. Comb the hair gently.

16. Use a hair dryer on the cool setting to dry hair, being very careful not to burn the scalp.

Tip **EASIER SHAMPOOING**
An enema bag attached to an IV pole provides an easy hose for shampooing.

Shaving

Shaving can be done by the person in your care, or you can shave his whiskers with a safety razor or an electric razor. If he wears dentures, make sure they are in his mouth. (See *One-Handed Tips*, p. 188.)

1. Assemble supplies—disposable gloves, safety razor, shaving cream, washcloth, towel, lotion.

2. Wash your hands.

3. Adjust the light so that you can clearly see his face but it is not shining in his eyes.

4. Spread a towel under his chin.

5. Soften the beard by wetting the face with a warm, damp washcloth.

6. Apply shaving cream to his face, carefully avoiding the eyes.

7. Hold the skin tight with one hand and using short firm strokes shave in the direction the hair grows.

8. Be careful of sensitive areas.

9. Rinse his skin with a wet washcloth.

10. Pat his face dry with the towel.

11. Apply lotion if the skin appears dry.

NOTE ▶ Never use an electric razor if the person is receiving oxygen.

Oral Care

Oral care includes cleaning the mouth and gums and the teeth or dentures. Always be patient and explain what you are about to do. (The person who refuses to brush his or her teeth can swish and spit out a fluoridated mouthwash rinse.) (📖 See *One-Handed Tips*, p. 188.)

1. Gather supplies—disposable gloves, a soft toothbrush, toothpaste or baking soda, warm water in a glass, dental floss, and a bowl.

2. Bring the person to an upright position.

3. If possible, allow the person to clean his or her own teeth. This should be done twice daily and after meals.

4. Be sure the person can spit out water before allowing a sip. Use a water glass for rinsing.

5. If necessary, ask the person to open his or her mouth. Gently brush the front and back teeth up and down.

6. Rinse well by having the person sip water and spit into a bowl.

Denture Cleaning

1. Remove the dentures from the mouth.

2. Run them under water and soak them in cleaner in a denture cup.

3. Rinse the person's mouth with water or mouthwash.

4. Stimulate (massage) the gums with a very soft toothbrush.

5. Return the dentures to the person's mouth.

 Even a person with dentures should have the soft tissues of the mouth checked regularly by a dentist.

Foot Care

For the comfort and good health of the person in your care:

- Provide properly fitting low-heeled shoes that close with Velcro® or elastic and have nonslip soles. Avoid shoes with heavy soles, running shoes with rubber tips over the toes, and shoes with thick cushioning.

- Provide cotton socks rather than acrylic.

- Trim the person's nails only after a bath when they have softened.

- Use a disposable sponge-tipped toothbrush to clean or dry between the toes.

- Check feet daily for bumps, cuts, and red spots.

Call the doctor or other health care provider if a sore develops on the foot. The person who is diabetic must have special foot care to prevent infections. Serious infections may result in the amputation of a foot.

 NOTE Foot pain can cause a person to lean back on the heels and increases the chance of a fall, so keep toenails trimmed and feet healthy.

Common Leg and Foot Problems and Solutions

Problem	Solution
Foot strain	Visit a podiatrist.
Calluses	Rub lanolin or lotion on the area; do not cut hard skin.
Cramps	Relieve by movement and massage.
Hammer toes and bunions	Wedge a pad between the big toe and the second toe to straighten them; cut holes in the shoe to relieve rubbing.
Leg ulcers (openings in the skin)	Follow the doctor's instructions. Exercise to keep the foot and ankle mobile.
Swollen legs	Follow the doctor's instructions for treatment of the underlying cause.
Varicose veins	Elevate the legs twice a day for 30 minutes. Before lowering the legs, apply an elastic bandage or stocking.

Dressing

Dressing a person with disabilities can be made easier by following a routine. Before you begin, lay the clothes out in the order in which they will be put on. (See *One-Handed Tips*, p. 188.)

- Dress the person while he or she is sitting.

- Use adaptive equipment like a button hook and shoe-horn. (See *Equipment and Supplies*, p. 142.)

- Use loose clothes that are easy to put on and have elastic waistbands, Velcro® fasteners, and front openings.

- Use bras that open and close in front.

- Use tube socks.

- Dress the weaker side first.

- For a person who is confined to bed, use a gown that closes in the back. This will make it easier when using a bedpan or urinal.

NOTE For a person who is confined to bed, be sure to smooth out all wrinkles in the clothes and bedding to prevent pressure sores.

Bed Making

Making a bed with someone in it will be easier if you follow these steps:

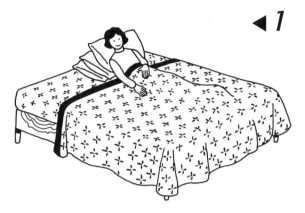

◀ 1
- The bed has two parts—the side the person is lying on and the side you are making.

- If you have a hospital bed, raise the height of the bed.

- Lower the head and foot of the bed so that it is flat.

Draw sheet

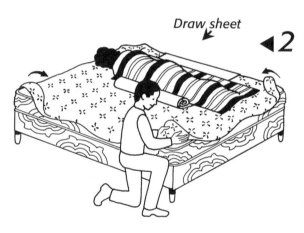

◀ 2
- Loosen the sheets on all sides.

- Remove the blankets and pillow, leaving only the bottom and top sheets.

- Cover the person with a bath blanket (a flannel sheet or large towel) for modesty and warmth.

- Pull the top sheet out from under the bath blanket.

- Raise the bed rail on the side across from you (the opposite side) so the person cannot fall out of bed. If you don't have a hospital bed, be sure the bed is pushed against the wall.

- Roll the person over to the opposite side of the bed.

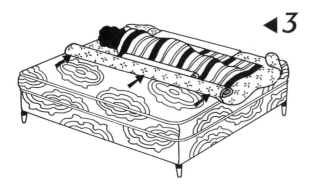

◀ 3
- Roll all the old bottom sheeting toward the person.

Clean sheet

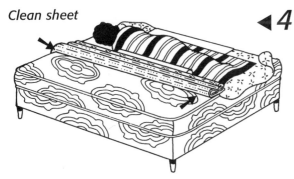

◀ 4
- Fold the clean sheet, along with other mattress covers, lengthwise.

- Place it on the bed with the middle fold running along the center of the mattress right beside the person's body.

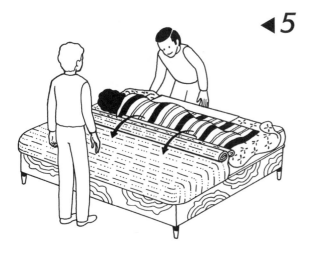

◀ 5
- Unfold the clean sheet and bring enough of it toward you to cover half of the bed.

- Gently lift the mattress and tuck the sheet in.

- Tuck the free edge of the draw sheet under the mattress on your side of the bed.

- Ask the person to roll over the linens in the middle of bed to the clean side.

OR

- Bend as close to the person's body as possible. Place your hand and arm under the person's shoulders and move the person and the bath blanket over the linens in the center of the bed.

- If it is a hospital bed, raise the bed rail on your side and lock it into place.

- Go to the other side and remove all soiled linen. Tuck in all the linen and pull tight on the sheets to remove all wrinkles so they don't rub and irritate the person's skin.

- Change the pillowcase.

- Spread the top sheet over the person and bath blanket.

- Ask the person to hold the sheet while you pull the bath blanket away.

- Tuck the sheet under the mattress at the foot of the bed.

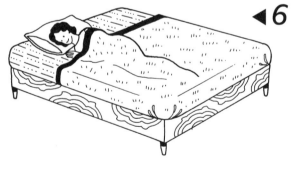

◀6
- Spread a blanket over the top. (The blanket should be up far enough to cover the person's shoulders.)

- Fold the sheet down over the blanket.

- Adjust the person in bed so he or she is comfortable.

Toileting

Always wear disposable gloves when helping with toileting. This prevents the spread of disease. Wash your hands before and after providing care.

Toileting in Bed

When a person is mobile, toileting in bed should not be encouraged.

Toileting in Bed for a Female or for Bowel Movements

1
- Warm the bedpan with warm water. Empty the water into the toilet.

- Powder the bedpan with talcum powder to keep the skin from sticking to it.

- Place a tissue or water in the pan to make cleaning easier. Or use a light spray of vegetable oil in the bedpan, which will make it easier to empty the contents.

- Raise the person's gown.

◀*2*
- Ask the person to raise her hips.

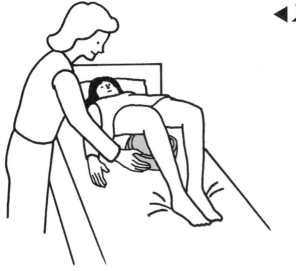

211

◄3   • If the person cannot raise her hips, turn her on her side and roll the hips back onto the bedpan.

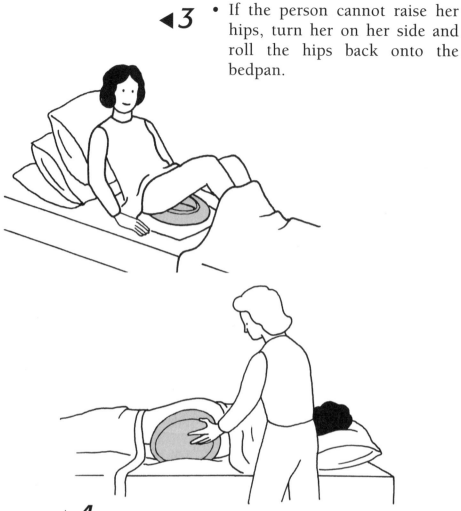

▲4

• If the person cannot do so, clean the anal area with bathroom tissue. Then use a wet tissue to clean the area.

• After the woman has urinated, pour a cup of warm water over her genitals and pat the area dry with a towel.

• Wash the person's hands.

• Remove and empty the bedpan.

• Be sure to wash your hands.

Using a Urinal

1. If the person can't do so himself, place the penis into the urinal as far as possible and hold it in.

2. When the person signals he is finished, remove and empty the urinal.

3. Wash his hands.

4. Wash your own hands.

Using a Commode

A portable commode is helpful for a person with limited mobility. The portable commode (with the pail removed) can be used over the toilet seat and as a shower seat.

Using a Portable Commode

1. Gather the portable commode, toilet tissue, a basin, a cup of water, a washcloth or paper towel, soap, and a towel.

2. Wash your hands.

3. Help the person onto the commode.

4. Offer toilet tissue when the person is finished.

5. Pour a cup of warm water on female genitalia.

6. Pat the area dry with a paper towel.

7. Offer a washcloth so the person can wash his or her hands.

8. Remove the pail from under the seat, empty it, rinse it with clear water, and empty the water into the toilet.

9. Wash your hands.

TOILET SAFETY
Use Velcro® with tape on the back and attach it to the back of the toilet or commode seat to keep the lid from falling.

Using the Bathroom Toilet

If the mobile person is missing the toilet, get a toilet seat in a color that is different from the floor color. This may help him see the toilet better. If he is failing to cleanse the anal area or failing to wash his hands, use tact to encourage him to do so. This will help prevent the spread of infections.

Catheters

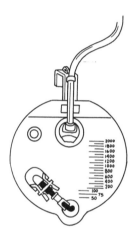

A urinary catheter is a device made from rubber or plastic that drains urine from the body. It is inserted by a nurse through the urethra (a tube that connects the bladder to the outside of the body) into the bladder (an organ that collects urine).

A Foley catheter stays in the bladder and drains into a bag that is attached to a person's leg, the bed, or a chair. When caring for someone with this kind of catheter (called an indwelling catheter), watch for these things:

1. Be sure the tube stays straight and drains properly. Check for kinks in the tubing.

2. Be sure the level of urine in the bag increases.

3. Be sure the drainage bag is always lower than the bladder.

4. Use tape or straps when securing a catheter to someone's inner thigh.

5. In males, an erection is a common effect when a catheter is inserted.

6. Tell the doctor if blood or sediment (matter that settles to the bottom) appears in the tubing or bag.

 A Foley catheter greatly increases the risk of infection. It is a last resort to manage incontinence (leaking of urine or inability to control bowel movements).

Care of the Person Who Has a Catheter

1. Wash your hands.

2. Put on disposable gloves.

3. Position the person on his or her back.

4. Take care not to pull on the catheter.

5. While holding the catheter, wash the area around it with a washcloth.

6. To avoid infection, wipe toward the anus, not back and forth.

 To prevent foul odors due to the growth of bacteria in the urine drainage bag, put a few drops of hydrogen peroxide in the bag when it is emptied.

Changing a Catheter from Straight Drainage to Leg Bag

1. Gather supplies—disposable gloves, a bed protector, alcohol wipes, and a leg bag with straps.

2. Uncover the end of the catheter and draining tubing; put a towel or other bed protector under this area.

3. Disconnect the drainage tubing from the catheter.

4. Wipe the attachment tube of the leg bag with an alcohol swab and insert it into the catheter.

5. Place the cap attached to the urinary drainage bag over the end of the tubing to keep it clean and prevent urine from leaking out.

6. Secure the tubing to the person's leg.

Condom Catheter

The doctor may prescribe a condom catheter for a male if infections from the indwelling catheter become a chronic problem. The catheter fits over the penis like a condom. Leakage is often a problem with this type of aid. **It is extremely important that a condom catheter not be secured too tightly, which can result in serious injury.** Other products for male incontinence are available that are less constricting, such as Bio Derm's Liberty Pouch, which uses "skin friendly" adhesive.

Incontinence

Incontinence is the leakage of urine or a bowel movement over which the person has no control. It can be a symptom of MS. In addition to bladder management medications, treatments can include bladder training, exercises to strengthen the pelvic floor (Kegel exercises), biofeedback, surgery, electrical muscle stimulator, urinary catheter, prosthetic devices, or external collection devices. Talk to the doctor about the options or treatments for the person in your care.

To Manage Incontinence:

- Avoid alcohol, coffee, spicy foods, and citrus foods. These can irritate the bladder and can increase the need to urinate.

- Give fluids at regular intervals to dilute the urine. This decreases the irritation of the bladder.

- Be sure the person in your care voids (goes to the bathroom) regularly, ideally every 2 to 3 hours. Use an alarm clock to keep track of the time.

- Provide clothing that can be easily removed.

- Keep a bedpan or a portable commode near the person.

- Provide absorbent products (adult diapers) to be worn under clothes.

- Stroke or tap the lower abdomen to cause voiding.

- Keep the skin dry and clean. Urine on the skin can cause pressure sores and infection.

- Your patience and understanding will help the person have confidence and self-respect.

 A precise diagnosis for incontinence must be made in order to come up with an effective treatment plan. If the primary care doctor and neurologist cannot solve the problem, see an experienced urologist familiar with MS.

Urinary Tract Infection

Urinary tract infection may be present if the person has any of the following signs or symptoms:

- blood in the urine

- a burning feeling when voiding

- cloudy urine with sediment (matter that settles to the bottom)

- pain in the lower abdomen or lower back

- fever and chills

- foul-smelling urine

- a frequent, strong urge to void or frequent voiding

Get in touch with the doctor if there is any sign of a urinary tract infection.

Optimal Bowel Function

Maintaining good bowel function can be a challenge, especially in individuals who are unable to get out of bed and get little exercise. For optimal bowel function—

- Set a time for bowel movements every day or every other day. The best time is 20–30 minutes after breakfast.

- Serve fruits, vegetables, and bran.

- Be sure the person in your care drinks 2 quarts (8 glasses) of water daily (or an amount directed by the doctor).

- Provide a chance for daily exercise.

- Use a stool softener or bulk agent if the stools are too hard. When using a bulk laxative, be sure that 6 to 8 glasses of water are taken per day. This will lessen the chance of severe constipation.

- Use glycerin suppositories as needed to help lubricate the bowels for ease of movement.

- Massage the abdomen in a clockwise direction. This can stimulate a bowel movement.

- Avoid laxatives and enemas unless specifically ordered by the doctor or nurse.

Diarrhea

Diarrhea (loose, watery stools) occurs when the intestines push stool along before the water in them can be reabsorbed (taken up) by the body. This condition can be caused by viral stomach flu, antibiotics, or other medications, or stress anxiety.

Diarrhea in people who are immobile is often caused by impaction. This is a blockage formed by hardened stool, with liquid stool passing around it. This must always be taken into consideration, because the usual treatments for diarrhea would be extremely dangerous if the diarrhea is being caused by impaction.

Hemorrhoids

Hemorrhoids are swollen inflamed veins around the anus. They cause tenderness, pain, and bleeding. To treat hemorrhoids, you should do the following:

- Be sure to keep anal area clean with premoistened tissues.

- Apply zinc oxide or petroleum jelly to the area.

- Relieve itching by using cold compresses on the anus for 10 minutes several times a day.

- Ask the doctor about suppositories.

Call the Doctor

- if blood from the hemorrhoids is dark red or brown and heavy

- if bleeding continues for more than one week

- if bleeding seems to occur for no reason

Control of Infection in the Home

Common health practices such as frequent hand-washing are necessary to avoid the risk of bacterial, viral, and fungal infections.

NOTE To minimize the chance of infection

- Always start with the cleanest area and work toward the dirtiest area.
- Always wash your hands before and after contact with the person in your care and with other people.
- Always wear disposable gloves when giving personal care.
- Always wash hands well when returning from a trip outside the house.
- Always wash your hands after using the toilet.

Cleaning Techniques

The following techniques will help cut the chance of infection in the home.

Caregiver Hand-washing

- Hand-washing is the single most effective way to prevent the spread of infection or germs.

- Use bottle-dispensed hand soap.

- If the person in your care has an infection, use antimicrobial soap.

- Rub your hands for at least 30 seconds to produce lots of lather. Do this away from running water so that the lather is not washed away.

- Use a nailbrush on your nails; keep nails trimmed.

- Wash front and back of hands, between fingers, and at least 2 inches up your wrists.

- Repeat the process.

- Dry your hands on a clean towel or a paper towel.

Handling Soiled Laundry

- Do not carry soiled linen close to your body.

- Never shake dirty items or put soiled linens on the floor. They can contaminate (infect) the floor and germs will be spread throughout the house on the soles of shoes.

- Store infected soiled linen in a leak-proof plastic bag and tie it closed.

- Bag soiled laundry in the same place it is used.

- Wash soiled linen separately from other clothes.

- Fill the machine with hot water, add bleach (no more than $1/4$ cup) and detergent. Rinse twice and then dry.

- Clean the washer by running it through a cycle with 1 cup of bleach or other disinfectant to kill germs.

- Use rubber gloves when handling soiled laundry.

- Wash your hands.

NOTE If urine is highly concentrated due to a bladder infection or dehydration, do not use bleach. The combination of ammonia in the urine and bleach can cause toxic fumes.

Sterilization

If you are sharing equipment with other members of the family, sterilizing will cut down on infection. If you are not sharing equipment, wiping it with a cotton ball soaked in alcohol is adequate.

Wet Heat Sterilization

1. Fill a large pot with water.

2. If sterilizing glass items, put a cloth in the bottom of the pot to prevent breakage.

3. Put items to be sterilized in the pot. These might include syringes, nail trimmers, and scissors.

4. Cover the pot and bring the water to a boil.

5. Boil, covered, for 20 minutes.

6. Leave the items in the pot until ready to use.

NOTE Cloth can be sterilized by holding a hot iron on it for a few seconds. Never use the microwave oven to disinfect (kill germs) any nonfood items. They can catch fire or explode.

Disposal of Body Fluids

- Wear disposable gloves (recommended for handling all body fluids).

- Flush liquid and solid waste down the toilet.

- Place used dressings and disposable (throwaway) pads in a sturdy plastic bag, tie securely, and place in a sealed container for collection.

Prevention of Odors Caused by Bacteria

Bacteria need moisture, warmth, oxygen, darkness, and nourishment to grow. Some strong odors may be eliminated by

- sprinkling baking soda on the wound dressing

- leaving an open can of finely ground coffee under the bed

- pouring a few drops of mouthwash in commodes and bedpans

- placing cotton balls soaked in mouthwash in the room

- spraying a fine mist of white distilled vinegar mixed with a few drops of eucalyptus or peppermint essential oil

- soaking cotton balls with vanilla extract and placing them in containers that hold on to strong odors

- using electrical and mechanical devices, such as plug-in air fresheners and fans, for removing odor

- buying natural organic room sprays

Skin Care and Prevention of Pressure Sores

Pressure sores (also called decubiti, or bedsores) are blisters or breaks in the skin. They are caused when the body's weight presses blood out of a certain area. The best treatment of pressure sores is prevention. How much time they take to heal depends on advanced they are.

Facts

- The most common areas for sores are the bony areas—tailbone, hips, heels, and elbows.

- Sores can appear when the skin keeps rubbing on a sheet.

- The skin breakdown starts from the inside, works up to the surface, and can happen in just 15 minutes.

- Damage can range from a change in color in unbroken skin to deep wounds down to the muscle or bone.

- For people with light skin in the first stage of a bedsore, the skin color may change to dark purple or red that does not turn pale under fingertip pressure. For people with dark skin, this area may become darker than normal.

- The affected area may feel warmer than the skin around it.

- Pressure sores that are not treated can lead to hospitalization and can require skin grafts.

Prevention

- Check the skin daily. (Bath time is the ideal time to do this.)

- Provide a well-balanced diet, with enough vitamin C, zinc, and protein.

- Keep the skin dry and clean (urine left on the skin can cause sores and infection).

- Keep clothing loose.

- If splints or braces are used, make sure they are adjusted properly.

- Massage the body with light pressure, using equal parts surgical spirit and glycerin. (Ask a nurse or a pharmacist for advice.)

- Turn a person who is unable to get out of bed at least every 2 hours. Change the person's positions. Smooth wrinkles out of sheets.

- Lightly tape foam to bony sections of the body using paper tape, which will not hurt the skin when peeled off.

- Use flannel or 100% cotton sheets to absorb moisture.

- Provide an egg-crate or sheepskin mattress pad for added comfort.

- Rent an electrically operated ripple bed. These beds have sections that can be inflated separately and at different times.

- Avoid using a plastic sheet or a Chux if they cause sweating.

- When the person is sitting, encourage changing the body position every 15 minutes.

- Use foam pads on chair seats to cushion the buttocks.

- Change the type of chair the person sits in; try an open-back garden chair occasionally.

- Provide as much exercise as possible.

WOUND PREVENTION

If a person tends to scratch or pick at a spot, have the person wear cotton gloves. (Make sure the hands are clean and dry before putting the gloves on.)

When Turning Someone in Bed to Minimize Sores:

1. Explain to the person what you are doing.

2. If possible, raise the bed to its highest position.

3. Lower the head of the bed to a flat position.

4. Loosen the draw sheet at the far side.

5. Stand in proper position as close to the person as possible.

6. Roll the far side of the draw sheet toward you and up close to the person's side.

7. Prop a pillow against the person's back.

8. Flex the person's knees slightly.

9. Place one pillow between the knees and another between the feet.

10. Check any catheter tubing.

Treatment

If you see pressure sores in your daily checking of the skin, you must alert the nurse or the doctor. General guidelines for treatment of these sores are as follows:

- To reduce the chance of infection, wear disposable gloves at all times when providing care.

- Take pressure off sores by changing the person's position often. Use pillows or a foam pad with at least 1 inch of padding to support the body.

- Do not position the person on his or her bony parts.

- Do not let the person lie on pressure sores.

- In bed, change the person's position at least every 2 hours.

- Follow the doctor's or nurse's treatment plan in applying medication to sores and bandaging the areas to protect them while they heal.

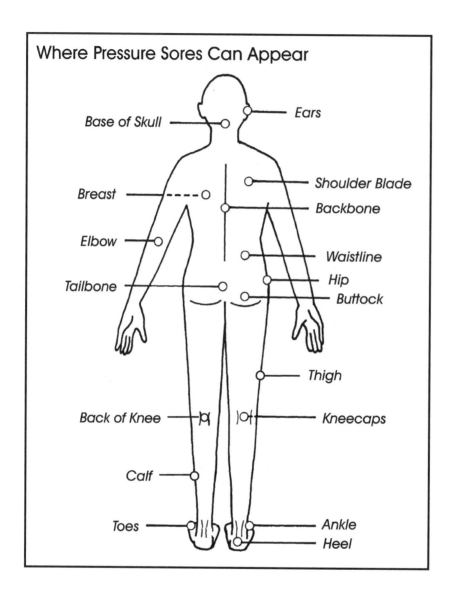

Where Pressure Sores Can Appear

Base of Skull

Ears

Breast

Shoulder Blade

Backbone

Elbow

Waistline

Tailbone

Hip

Buttock

Thigh

Back of Knee

Kneecaps

Calf

Toes

Ankle

Heel

Eating

Mealtimes are important because they provide a welcome break in the day. If it is not too distracting for the person in your care, meals can be eaten with the family. It is important that mealtimes be enjoyable so that the person will look forward to eating. (See *One-Handed Tips*, p. 188.)

Look for these free or low-cost solutions:

Community meals—local meal programs sponsored by the federal government and open to those over 59 and their spouses. Call the local Area Agency on Aging or Department of Health and Human Resources.

Meals-on-Wheels—hot meals delivered to the home. Call the Visiting Nurse Association.

Food stamps—help based on income that can stretch food dollars. Call the Department of Health and Human Resources or the Area Agency on Aging.

For best results at mealtime:

- Allow 30 to 45 minutes for eating.

- Avoid fussy meal presentation.

- Make sure all items are ready to eat and within reach.

- Provide a comfortable table and chair or other eating arrangement.

- Supply easy-to-hold eating utensils. To avoid cuts, throw out all chipped cups and plates.

- Reduce excess noise such as TV and radio.

- If the person's vision is poor, place the same foods in the same spot on the plate every time.

Feeding Someone in Bed

1. Prop the head with pillows.

2. Provide an over-the-bed table.

3. Do not rush feeding, but maintain a steady pace.

4. Cut the food into bite-size portions.

5. Fill cups only halfway.

6. Let the person hold the cup if he or she wants to. (A terry cloth tennis wristband slipped over the cup may make it easier to hold.)

7. Use available eating aids. (📖 See *Equipment and Supplies,* p. 129.)

8. Keep a moist hand towel to wipe the person's mouth and hands gently. The chains used to hang eyeglasses around the neck can be used to hold a napkin in place.

FEEDING IN BED

An adjustable ironing board may be used as an over-the-bed table for activities or eating.

Feeding the Person Who Is Disabled

1. Name the food being offered.

2. If the person plays with food, limit the choices being offered. (Playing with food occurs because a person is confused and unable to make choices.)

3. Check the temperature of the food often.

4. Be gentle with forks and spoons. (A rubber-tipped baby spoon may be helpful.)

5. Feed at a steady pace, alternating food with drink.

6. Remove a spoon from the person's mouth very slowly. If the person clenches the spoon, let go of it and wait for the jaw to relax.

7. Give simple instructions such as "Open your mouth," "Move your tongue," "Now swallow."

8. If the person spits food out, try feeding later.

9. If the person refuses food, provide a drink and return in 10 minutes with the food tray.

10. Between meals, provide a nourishing snack, such as stewed fruit, tapioca pudding, or finger foods.

Boosting Food Intake When the Appetite Is Poor

- Offer more food at the time of day when the person is most hungry or less tired.

- To increase the appeal of food for those with decreased taste and smell, provide strong flavors.

- Use milk or cream instead of water in soups and cooked cereal.

- Add fat by using butter, margarine, or olive oil on foods.

- Add nonfat dry-milk powder to foods like yogurt, mashed potatoes, gravy, and sauces.

- Tell the person to eat with his or her fingers if that is the only way to get the person to eat.

- Offer milk or fruit shakes.

- Offer puréed (finely ground) baby foods.

(See *Diet, Nutrition, and Exercise*, p. 269.)

Eating Problems and Solutions

Drooling—Use a straw if possible; help close the mouth with your hand. (However, sometimes the use of a straw can cause choking if liquid touches the back of the mouth too quickly.)

Spitting out food—Ask the doctor if the cause is moodiness or disease.

Too much swallowing or chewing—Coach the person to alternate hot and cold bites.

Difficulty chewing—Change the diet to soft foods.

Difficulty swallowing—Put foods through a blender or food mill; avoid thin liquids and instead serve thick liquids such as milk shakes.

Poor scooping—Use bowls instead of plates.

Difficulty cutting food—Use a small pizza cutter or rolling knife.

Trouble moving food to the back of the mouth—Change the food's thickness and demonstrate how to direct the food to the center of the mouth.

Too dry or too wet mouth—Ask the doctor or the pharmacist if this is a side effect of medications.

Too easily distracted—Pull down the shades and remove the distractions.

NOTE Difficulty in swallowing can cause food or liquids to be taken into the lungs, which can lead to pneumonia. Reduce the chance of food entering the lungs by keeping the person upright for at least 30 minutes after a meal.

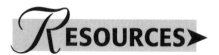

RESOURCES

Meeting Life's Challenges
9042 Aspen Grove Lane
Madison, WI 53717
Fax (608) 824-0403
www.meetinglifeschallenges.com
E-mail: help@meetinglifeschallenges.com
Offers a guide called Dressing Tips and Clothing Resources for Making Life Easier, *by Shelley P. Schwarz, a guide to dressing for people with disabilities plus more than 100 resources for custom clothing.*

National Association for Continence (NAFC)
P.O. Box 8310
Spartanburg, SC 29305-8310
(800) 252-3337; (864) 579-7900; Fax (864) 579-7902
www.nafc.org
NAFC is a leading source of education and support to the public about the diagnosis, treatments, and management alternatives for incontinence.

If you don't have home access to the Internet, ask your local library to help you locate any Web site.

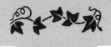

Therapies

Therapies

The following information is provided for your general knowledge. It IS NOT a substitute for training with professional therapists.

Physical Therapy

What a Physical Therapist Does

A physical therapist treats a person to relieve pain, build up and restore muscle function, and maintain the best possible performance. The therapist does this by using physical means such as active and passive exercise, massage, heat, water, and electricity. Broadly speaking, a physical therapist:

- sets up the goals of treatment with patient and family
- shows how to use special equipment
- instructs in routine daily functions
- teaches safe ways to move
- sets up and teaches an exercise program

 NOTE The American Physical Therapy Association, often located in the state capital, can provide a list of licensed therapists.

What a Physical Therapist Determines

Depending on a person's physical condition, a therapist may work on range-of-motion exercises, correct body positions when resting, devices to help the person in your care, and other simple ways to improve daily functions.

A physical therapist checks things that can affect a person's daily activities—

- the person's attitude toward his situation

- how well he can move his muscles and joints (range of motion)

- his ability to see, smell, hear, and feel

- what he can do on his own and what he needs to learn

- his equipment needs, now and in the future

- what can be improved in the home to make moving around safer and more comfortable

- who can and will help to give support

Range-of-Motion (ROM) Exercises

The purpose of range-of-motion exercises is to relieve pain, maintain normal body alignment (positions), help prevent skin swelling and breakdown, and promote bone formation. A ROM exercise program should be started before deformities develop. Here are some things to do when you are asked to help with exercises at home:

- Communicate what you are doing.

- Use the flats of both hands, not the fingertips, to hold a body part.

- Take each movement only as far as the joint will go into a comfortable stretch. (Mild discomfort is okay, but it should go away quickly.)

Joints Used in ROM

▲ shoulder

▲ hip

▲ shoulders

▲ finger/thumb

▲ feet, ankle, toe

▲ hands

▲ wrists

▲ elbows

▲ neck

- Do each exercise 3 to 5 times.

- Use slow steady movements to help relax muscles and increase joint range.

- If joints are swollen and painful, exercise very gently.

Proper Positions to Use When Resting:

- flat on the back or no more than 30° raised

- prone (lying flat) on the stomach (for up to 20 to 30 minutes only, not for sleeping)

- one-quarter left or right turn onto the back

- three-quarters right or left turn on to the stomach

- aided by special positioning devices (for example, splints for leg, foot, hand, or back support)

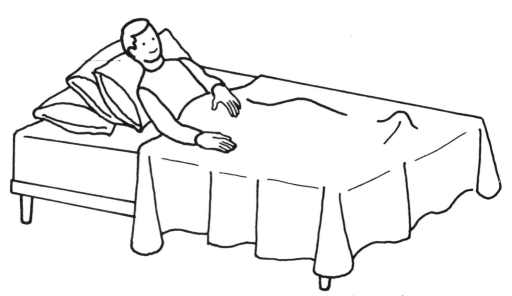

▲ *When resting keep head elevated no more than 30 degrees.*

Occupational Therapy

Occupational therapy is designed to help people regain and build skills that are important for functioning on their own. The occupational therapist will help the person evaluate levels of function.

The occupational therapist will—

- test a person's strength, range of motion, endurance (the ability to continue an activity or effort), and dexterity (skill in using hands) to do everyday tasks that were done easily before an illness or injury happened

- design a program of activities and solutions that ensure the greatest possible independence

- provide training to relearn everyday activities of daily living like eating, grooming, dressing, toileting, bathing, and leisure activities

- decide whether special equipment is needed, such as wheelchairs, feeding devices, transfer equipment, hand and skin devices

- help the stroke survivor fight tiredness and problems with thinking

Speech Therapy

Speech therapy is the treatment of disorders that involve speaking, hearing, writing, reading, and other communication required for the activities of daily living. Speech therapists also teach people to swallow foods and liquids safely.

A speech therapist or speech pathologist works to—

- strengthen weakened oral muscles through exercises

- teach methods of basic communication

- teach a patient and family how to manage a communication or swallowing disorder

Acupuncture

Acupuncture is one form of treatment in traditional Chinese medicine. It is based on the theory that the energy flows in channels or meridians in the body. Acupuncturists alter the flow of energy by inserting thin, disposable, metallic needles into points along the energy meridians (or pathways). Similar methods including finger pressure, cupping with small heated cups, and electroacupuncture with electrically stimulated needles use the same acupuncture points.

Acupuncture is a safe treatment for stroke survivors. The needles are essentially painless and are well tolerated by most people. Survivors often report relief from long-term symptoms, such as pain, spasticity (spasm), numbness and tingling, bladder problems, and depression. It is important to remember that acupuncture must be combined with standard medical treatment. Also, the effect of acupuncture on the body's immune system is not clear.

Pet Therapy

A cat, bird, or dog can bring great joy to people. They provide companionship, relaxation, and a chance to exercise. They also lessen the boredom and fear caused by loneliness.

- Before selecting a dog, check canine-assistant programs in your area. Dogs that were rejected from the program may be ideal for the person in your care.

- Choose a mature dog that is housetrained; do not get a puppy.

- Have a dog or cat neutered or spayed to lessen the chance of roaming.

- Keep up all pet vaccinations.

- Never clean pet cages or feeding dishes in the kitchen sink.

 NOTE Be aware that animals carry bacteria and intestinal parasites. Individuals with weakened immune systems should not change the litter box or pick up outside waste and should wash their hands frequently.

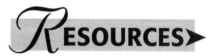

Acufinder.com
(760) 630-3600
www.acufinder.com
A referral service that lists state-licensed acupuncturists.

American Academy of Medical Acupuncture
(800) 521-2262
www.medicalacupuncture.org

Delta Society
875 124th Ave NE, Suite 101
Bellevue, WA 98005
(425) 226-7357; Fax (425) 235-1076
www.deltasociety.org
E-Mail: info@deltasociety.org
Provides information on the human–animal bond and information on how to obtain a service animal.

National Center of Complementary and Alternative Medicine Clearinghouse
(888) 644-6226
www.nccam.nih.gov

Contact your local **Humane Society** for information about pet therapy.

If you don't have home access to the Internet, ask your local library to help you locate any Web site.

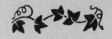

Special Challenges

Special Challenges

*C*ommunication is the ability to speak, understand speech, read, write, and motion with the hands. Non-verbal messages are expressed through silence, body movements, or the look on someone's face. Be aware that words can carry one message, the body another.

Communication Changes After Stroke

Loss of Speech in Stroke Patients

Loss of speech can happen due to damage to the brain or lack of oxygen. The person who experiences such a loss still has the same intelligence he or she had before the injury, though this fact may be hard to remember in light of dramatic changes in behavior.

- The communication problem may involve talking or understanding.

- The person may be able to say words at one time and then not at another, or may repeat the same word over and over.

- The person may unknowingly swear or laugh or cry frequently.

- Left-brain damage affects listening, speaking, reading, and writing.

- Right-brain damage affects non-linguistic skills such as assessing a situation and behaving appropriately, controlling facial expressions, and understanding tones of voice.

A speech therapist can suggest specific tasks to help the person communicate—for example,

- using pictures instead of words
- teaching specific exercises to strengthen the muscles of the face, lips, or tongue.

To communicate better with the stroke survivor, try:

- getting the person's attention by lightly touching her arm before speaking
- speaking slowly and simply
- asking questions that require simple yes/no answers
- providing opportunities for the person to hear speech
- helping the person communicate frustrations
- pacing activities, because the person will tire easily
- not allowing the person to become bossy

Aphasia

Survivors of left-brain strokes often have communication problems. The most common of these is a loss of language function caused by the stroke, affecting the ability to speak or comprehend speech and the ability to read or write. This is called "aphasia."

NOTE Aphasia is a problem with **language,** not cognitive ability. A person with aphasia can think and reason as he always did, but he cannot **express** those thoughts (expressive aphasia) or **comprehend** the expression of others (receptive aphasia). For this reason, it may be extremely distressing to both survivor and family.

Aphasia can be so severe that communication is impossible, or it may be very mild, such as occasional difficulty finding the right word. It may affect a single aspect of language use, such as the ability to retrieve the names of things. More often it involves multiple aspects of communication.

Tips for Communicating with a Survivor with Aphasia

No two people with aphasia are alike with respect to severity, former speech and language skills, or personality. But it is essential for your survivor to communicate as successfully as possible from the very beginning of the recovery process. Here are some suggestions to improve communication:

- Make sure you have your survivor's attention before communicating.

- During conversation, minimize or eliminate background noise (television, radio, other people) as much as possible.

- Keep communication simple but adult, **don't use baby talk**. Simplify your sentences and reduce your rate of speech. Don't speak louder than normal but emphasize key words. Don't "talk down" to the person with aphasia.

- Encourage and use other modes of communication (writing, drawing, yes/no responses, choices, gestures, eye contact, facial expressions) in addition to speech.

- Have a pencil and paper handy.

- Accept any form of communication as equally valid: gestures, writing, drawing, using a communication notebook, or speech.

- When you are talking, provide the listener with words or phrases that help explain the meaning of what is being communicated, especially if switching subjects:

"I want to talk about the stroke support group meeting now." This primes the listener to listen for certain words.

- Give your survivor time to talk and let him have a reasonable time to respond. Avoid speaking for the person with aphasia except when necessary and ask permission before doing so.

- Praise all attempts to speak; make speaking a pleasant experience and provide stimulating conversation. Downplay errors and avoid frequent corrections. Every word doesn't have to be perfect.

- Add gestures and visual aids to your communication whenever possible. Repeat a statement when necessary.

- Create an atmosphere in which your survivor is encouraged to make decisions, offer comments, and communicate thoughts and desires.

- Encourage the person in your care to be as independent as possible. Avoid being overprotective.

- Whenever possible, continue normal activities (such as dinner with family, company, going out). Do not shield people with aphasia from family or friends or ignore them in a group conversation. Rather, try to involve them in family decision-making as much as possible.

- Be a communication partner, not a therapist. At least once a day have a pleasant conversation with the person in your care.

These guidelines will enhance communication with a person who has aphasia. However, improvements may not be immediate or dramatic.

> *Tip* Restoring language fluency and word-finding ability takes time, so be patient and encourage patience in your survivor. Improvement can't happen without practice. Keep the person in your care involved with language by going places; also encourage reading, writing, and speaking.

Technology May Help

There have been many advances in speech therapy, especially in the use of computer programs to deliver speech therapy at home. In addition, there are many augmentative communication devices, which means technology that is used to improve whatever communication capability a person has. Evaluation by a speech-language pathologist will assure that you get the right device or software.

> *Tip* The American Speech/Language and Hearing Association (ASHA) has produced a booklet to help you decide when a communication-improving device such as a hearing aide will help enhance communication. For a free copy of "Augmentative Communication for Consumers," contact the American Speech-Language-Hearing Association (ASHA), Phone: 800-638-8255 or 301-987-5700; http://www.asha.org/

Driving After Stroke

Beyond convenience and necessity, driving is important for a feeling of independence. Unfortunately, stroke can affect the areas of the brain that control the abilities necessary for driving, from perception and decision-making to reflexes and motor control. The ability to react quickly may be lost. Peripheral vision may be limited.

Paralysis, partial paralysis or weakness, and difficulty coordinating muscle movement (spasticity and ataxia) are some of the stroke conditions that can make it difficult to drive safely.

Because of these problems, driving after a stroke may be dangerous. Survivors and caregivers should carefully consider whether it would be safe for the survivor to drive again.

Safety is the primary concern, so it's important for you to be able to spot the signals that indicate driving may be unsafe. The American Stroke Association has identified these warning signs. Driving is dangerous when the survivor—

- drives too fast or too slow for road conditions or posted speeds

- needs help or instructions from passengers

- doesn't observe signs or signals

- makes slow or poor decisions about distance

- gets easily frustrated or confused

- gets lost often, even in familiar areas

- has accidents or close calls

- drifts across lane markings into other lanes

NOTE Survivors may have difficulty noticing any difference in their driving ability since their stroke, even if the warning signs are obvious to others. Don't expect them to agree immediately to give up the keys.

If driving is determined to be a possibility for your survivor, here are some suggestions as to what to do to next.

- First step, talk to an occupational therapist. She can provide up-to-date information and a professional opinion on the survivor's capabilities.

- Next, contact your state's Department of Motor Vehicles (DMV). Ask for the office of driver safety to get the requirements for survivors who want to drive.

- Finally, have your survivor tested. Professionals such as driver rehabilitation specialists can perform a reliable assessment of driving ability. A typical test will evaluate perception, functional ability, reaction time, and performance behind the wheel. Depending on your state's laws, your survivor may need to apply for a new driver's license.

 Tip When a survivor has completed physical and occupational rehab but still hasn't regained his or her driving abilities, a driver-retraining program may help. These programs can provide driving assessments, classroom instruction, and suggestions for modifying a vehicle with adaptive equipment. Check with your local rehab center or contact the Adaptive Driving Alliance (623-434-0722 or www.adamobility.com) to locate a program in your area.

Adapting a Vehicle

Your survivor may be able to drive safely if his vehicle is properly adapted. Some adaptive innovations include:

- A spinner knob for the steering wheel, which enables one-handed driving (Check with the DMV to make sure it's legal to use a knob in your state.)

- A left-foot gas pedal for survivors who cannot use their right foot

- Hand controls
- Wheelchair lifts and restraint systems for minivans

Tip If your vehicle needs modifying, research costs and ask dealers about financial assistance programs. Nonprofit agencies sometimes offer grants to pay for modifications, and some health-insurance plans and workers' compensation programs offer financial assistance. Check with your state's department of vocational rehabilitation.

Once the vehicle is adapted, there are training requirements for operating an adapted vehicle. The equipment provider typically gives information on the use of your adapted vehicle, but the survivor will also need instruction from a qualified driving rehabilitation specialist. To locate a specialist in your area, contact the Association for Driver Rehabilitation Specialists at 1-800-290-2344 or www.aded.net.

Returning to Work After Stroke

For many stroke survivors, returning to work is the gold standard by which they measure their recovery. Younger survivors with children still at home may feel they have to help support a family. Survivors closer to retirement age may work because for them a job is more than money—it's self-esteem.

Survivors of working age don't easily give up on their careers. This is a common reaction. Survivors often judge their recovery status by their success in the structured and routine environment of therapy, but the work world is more complex and demanding.

> *Tip* A survivor's awareness of changed abilities can be limited by the damage done by the stroke. Family members and therapists may be more aware of the survivor's functional losses and their implications, while the survivor minimizes or denies problems.

Eager to return to work, survivors often fail to judge the everyday demands of a job, things like having adequate energy, getting along with others, the pace, and the flexibility of thought needed to make independent decisions. Coming from rehab, they may fail to appreciate these complicating factors.

Improvement generally begins by gaining a better understanding of the consequences of the stroke and its affects on behavior. It helps when the survivor understands the potential for recovery and its rate. Opportunities for rehabilitation therapy and home-therapy programs offer the chance for additional recovery. They allow survivors to experience their current skills and provide critical feedback about their new self.

NOTE Your state's vocational rehab department is the place to start the search for employment after stroke. They can do assessments, provide guidance on workplace accommodations, and evaluate what kind of retraining is necessary.

It will help you help your survivor if you understand that it is unlikely that she will return to a previous job.

Choosing a career path that matches your survivor's post-stroke strengths is a key component of successfully returning to work.

In most cases, survivors must undergo some form of retraining. Since education is the key to returning to work, many states pay for at least part of the cost, but usually do not pay for transportation and living expenses.

When returning to school, contact the office of disability accommodations. They will work out accommodations that may include time-and-a-half on tests, extra tutoring, tape recording of lectures, and release from foreign language requirements. Other accommodations may be available.

Survivors returning to work often misjudge how much energy it takes to work full time. Nor do they realistically appreciate the pace and accuracy required by most jobs. You can increase the odds of your survivor's success by discussing what will happen once he returns to work. This can help when things are not as easy or take much more time than he imagines they will. It allows you to discuss the possible scenarios that may come up at work and ways of coping with them.

> **Tip** Survivors wanting to return to work should consider starting with part-time volunteer activities. These efforts can provide realistic feedback about the survivor's stamina and emotional state.

Steps Necessary to Return to Work

Step 1: Have the survivor assessed.

Just because your survivor wants to return to work doesn't mean she is ready. There may be psychological problems, as well as other predictable obstacles, like housing, finances, transportation, medical and medication requirements.

When survivors can't return to their previous jobs, it is a blow to their self-esteem. Counseling from a therapist or clergy can help. It may also help to get career counseling from the state rehab agency or a nonprofit disability organization. A career counselor can develop a plan for achieving specific goals.

Step 2: The survivor needs a mentor.

A mentor is someone who is honest, objective, and supportive. This person may be a counselor, another disabled person who has succeeded in returning to work, a teacher, or clergy. Their job is to give honest feedback and consistent encouragement.

Step 3: The survivor must decide what he wants to do.

People often find that the direction of their lives changes after stroke. Sometimes that comes as a result of physical or cognitive limitations. People commonly have new insights about themselves and their purpose as a result of the introspection that often follows a life-threatening experience. Sometimes they find that overcoming a disability is specialized job training for the work they want to do. Physical, cognitive, and speech changes that accompany stroke may require a career change.

> *Tip*
>
> Relationships become increasingly important to people who have survived a health crisis, they mean much more than specific jobs and titles. Creating those relationships may be the most important thing, and that can be fulfilled through work or volunteer settings, or through family or spiritual pursuits.

Step 4: The survivor needs a plan.

Whether or not someone has a disability, getting a job is rarely easy or comfortable. The process is made easier by a detailed plan of what is needed and how to get it. A career counselor who works with disabled people should be able to provide a roadmap to help your survivor achieve her goals.

Step 5: The survivor will likely need education.

Not surprisingly, a new career generally requires new training or further education. In most states, the rehab agency can help survivors pay for educational and training services. They may pay all the costs or only part, but they are the first place you should investigate. The rehab agency should also be able to guide you in evaluating the kinds of accommodations offered by different schools.

Step 6: The survivor may need to modify expectations.

For many survivors, full-time employment is unrealistic—there may just be too much stress in a 40-hour week. Coming home exhausted every day is not sustainable and will create health complications. Part-time work or volunteer activities may be more realistic, especially to start. Counseling may be necessary to uncouple work and self-esteem in your survivor's mind.

Step 7: Finally, both of you must get busy networking.

Networking is essential to finding a job, but before a network can work, your survivor has to be clear about what he or she wants. Experts say that people rarely find a job in their first four levels of networking. In other words, you may have to meet a lot of people before you get to the person who has the job. And remember, the majority of jobs are never listed in the newspaper or any other public place. About the only way to find out about those jobs is to know somebody who knows somebody. Another way is through a temporary agency. Online job databases like www.monster.com and www.careerone stop.org may be helpful as well. Volunteer activities also expand your survivor's network of contacts.

 Tip Rather than ask the people in your network if they know about any jobs, ask instead if they know anybody in the field you are interested in or who works at a company in that business. Make it your goal to get the name and contact information of at least one person in the field your survivor is interested in from every person you talk to about the job search.

Americans with Disability Act (ADA)

Despite the ADA, prejudice against people with disabilities is a big obstacle. The ADA gives a legal remedy to disabled people who are discriminated against as a result of their disability. The legislation requires employers to make "reasonable accommodation" to help a disabled worker do his or her job. It does not require them to do *everything* possible to accommodate a disability.

Tip The Job Accommodation Network is a federally funded consulting service that provides both high- and low-tech solutions for adapting work environments for persons with disabilities. Call 800-526-7234 or 877-781-9403 (V/TTY) worldwide. http://janweb.icdi.wvu.edu/

The reality of the workplace is that employers continue to discriminate against disabled people. The search for meaningful employment may be long and emotionally trying for you and your survivor. You will both weather this time better if you have a support network of family, friends, or a stroke support group who know what's going on. A mentor's #1 job is encouragement. So is the caregiver's!

Tip Studies indicate that people with a disability who have the most success in returning to work either enter a small or family-owned business, work in childcare or out of their homes, and only work part time.

Stroke families often make big sacrifices while their survivors come to terms with their disabilities, learning ways to overcome the challenges they face, and then finding a place for themselves in an ever-changing economy. On this journey, there will be highs and lows, moments of joy, and dashed expectations. It may help you and your survivor deal with the frustration, anger, and confusion that arise if you remember that *breakthroughs* are almost always preceded by *breakdowns*. The race often goes to those who persist—DON'T GIVE UP!

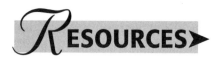

RESOURCES

Adaptive Driving Alliance
(633) 434-0722
www.adamobility.com

For information on the **Americans with Disabilities Act**, type "ADA" into your search engine. This will take you to the home page.

American Occupational Therapy Association
4720 Montgomery Lane
P.O, Box 31220
Bethesda, MD 20824-1220
(301) 652-2682
Fax (301) 652-7711
(800) 377-8555 TDD
www.aota.org/olderdriver/

American Speech/Language Association
(800) 638-TALK (8255)
www.asha.org

Aphasia Hope Foundation
(866) 449-5804
www.aphasiahope.org

Association of Driver Rehabilitation Specialists
(800) 290-2344
www.aded.net

National Aphasia Association
(800) 922-4NAA (4622)
www.aphasia.org

National Highway Safety Administration
(888) 327-4236
www.nhtsa.dot.gov (type "stroke" in the search window)
Free pamphlet of particular interest: "Driving When You Have Had a Stroke."

If you don't have home access to the Internet, ask your local library to help you locate any Web site.

Diet, Nutrition, and Exercise

Diet, Nutrition, and Exercise

A person's quality of life can often be improved by focusing on those aspects of health that can be changed. Good health has a lot to do with what you do each and every day. Eating right and being physically active are areas in which you can be in control. The lifestyle habits you choose can have a lot to do with feeling good today and staying healthy tomorrow.

Diet and Exercise Contribute to Stroke Risk

Almost certainly your survivor returned home with diet and exercise "prescriptions." Poor diet and lack of exercise contribute to stroke and other cardiovascular diseases in several ways:

1. Diet affects dietary cholesterol, which has a major impact on atherosclerosis. High cholesterol dramatically increases the risk of all cardiovascular diseases, including ischemic stroke.

2. Diet affects blood pressure. High blood pressure dramatically increases the risk of stroke and other cardiovascular disease.

3. Diet impacts diabetes, and diabetes dramatically increases the risk of stroke and cardiovascular disease.

4. Diet contributes to overweight and obesity, which in turn increases the risk of diabetes and cardiovascular disease. It also increases the risk of depression, which increases stroke risk.

5. Exercise *positively* affects both obesity and blood pressure, decreasing the risk of stroke and cardiovascular disease.

> **NOTE** The diet and exercise prescriptions your doctor gave your survivor are as important as the medication prescriptions given.

Weight Loss

This is not a diet book, but if you or your survivor is overweight, then losing weight will require some change in diet. Whatever diet your doctor recommends, losing weight is a matter of taking in fewer calories than your body burns. It's like balancing a caloric checkbook, where calories are cash and weight is savings.

More calories burned than eaten = decreasing weight

More calories eaten than burned = increasing weight

> **NOTE** If you eat 10 calories more than you burn every day for a year, you'll gain 1 lb—3,600 calories = 1 lb.
>
> If you do that for 20 years—just 10 calories more a day—at the end of 20 years, you'll have gained 20 lbs.
>
> Ten calories is an insignificant amount of food. For many people, the overage is more in the hundreds-of-calories range. This simple equation may explain why 60 percent of Americans are either overweight or obese.

Diet and Nutrition Education

If you need reliable, well-organized, user-friendly advice about a healthy diet, get a copy of *The No-Fad Diet* from the American Heart Association (AHA). It is the only diet book the AHA has ever written, and it contains all the information you need about diet, exercise, and behavior change. It also contains sample meal plans, easy-to-prepare recipes, and information on starting an exercise program. One of the key features of the book is that it addresses the psychological component of changing behavior. The book is available at the American Stroke Association Web site, through online booksellers, or your local bookstore. In addition, AHA offers many cookbooks, all designed to combat cardiovascular disease and stroke.

Cholesterol

Cholesterol is present in the cell wall of every cell in animal bodies, including human animals. The amount of cholesterol determines how permeable (leaky) the cell is. Cholesterol has a couple of other positive roles, but that cell-wall function is the main one. Cholesterol is so important to our basic biology that our bodies manufacture all the cholesterol they need from saturated fat. Dietary cholesterol is extra.

 Cholesterol manufacture is under genetic control, and it is possible that diet and exercise won't be enough to lower your survivor's numbers. Cholesterol-lowering medication may be called for. Older cholesterol drugs work to block absorption of dietary cholesterol. A new type of drug addresses the manufacture of cholesterol in the liver.

Tip Lowering the intake of *saturated fat* will help lower cholesterol level.

Saturated fat is fat that is solid at room temperature, like butter or the fat on meat.

Unsaturated fat is liquid at room temperature, like vegetable oil.

To get from your liver to your cells, cholesterol has to travel in your blood. Although technically a kind of fat, cholesterol is like a wax, think egg-yolk residue on a plate after breakfast. Since blood is mostly water, it doesn't know what to do with wax. It can't dissolve it, so it wraps it in protein. That's where cholesterol gets its other name—lipoprotein.

Tip Baffled by the LDL/HDL distinction? Low-density lipoprotein (LDL) is *bad* cholesterol, think L for "lousy." Another easy way to remember this is to think of LDL as "less-desirable lipids." LDL cholesterol doesn't move in liquid as well and tends to be stickier and so sticks to blood-vessel walls. High-density lipoprotein (HDL) is the *good* kind, think H for "healthy" or HDL as "highly desirable lipids." HDL tends to flow more freely in the blood stream and is not as sticky.

Whether cholesterol is LDL or HDL is largely determined by activity levels—in other words, you can't eat more or less of either one. To increase HDL levels exercise more.

To reduce your survivor's dietary cholesterol will require you to alter his or her intake of animal products. All meat, dairy, and eggs contain some cholesterol, no matter their fat content, because *all* animal cells contain cholesterol.

In addition, tropical oils (palm and coconut) and partially hydrogenated oils also contribute to cholesterol numbers.

Tip Partially hydrogenated oil is vegetable oil with hydrogen whipped into it, generally to increase shelf life. Nutritionists now label these oils as "trans-fat." It is suspected that trans-fats also contribute to atherosclerosis (a disease in which cholesterol deposits form on the walls of arteries, narrowing them).

Blood Pressure

Diet affects blood pressure because it affects weight, sodium, and atherosclerosis. Atherosclerosis increases blood pressure by narrowing arteries from the inside. Sodium causes water retention because our kidneys need water to maintain a proper electrolyte balance. This retained water puts pressure on the blood vessels and keeps them from relaxing, thereby increasing blood pressure.

Nutrition scientists have formulated the DASH Diet. (DASH stands for **d**ietary **a**pproach to **s**top **h**ypertension.) The DASH Diet was designed by the National Heart, Lung and Blood Institute after rigorous investigation into which vitamins, minerals, and micronutrients affected blood pressure.

The DASH Diet is low in saturated fat, cholesterol, and total fat. It emphasizes fruits, vegetables, and low-fat dairy foods, and includes whole-grain products, fish, poultry, and nuts. It is reduced in red meat, sweets, and sugar-containing beverages, and is rich in magnesium, potassium, and calcium, as well as protein and fiber. It controls for sodium. Research has reported reductions in blood pressure in as little as two weeks after beginning the DASH diet.

Facts about the DASH Eating Plan is a 24-page booklet that includes a week's worth of recipes. It is published by the National Institutes of Health, NIH Publication 03-4082, May 2003. E-mail nhlbi@prospectassoc.com or call 301-592-8573. To view online, go to www.nhlbi.nih.gov and type the booklet's title in the search window.

 Blood pressure is affected by more than one biological/chemical mechanism. In order to control high blood pressure, doctors may prescribe more than one blood pressure medication because different drugs work with different mechanisms. Each pill plays a role in reducing the numbers, as does your diet.

A Foundation of Good Nutrition

Bringing good nutrition to the table takes planning, attention, and some imagination. A foundation to healthy eating can be found in the U.S. Department of Agriculture's *MyPyramid*. Making smart choices from each part of the pyramid is the best way to ensure one's body gets the balanced nutrition it needs. Here are some easy tips to make the most of every food group, and get the most from the calories eaten:

- **Focus on fruits.** Select fresh, frozen, canned, or dried over juices for most of your fruit choices.

- **Vary your vegetables.** Choose from a rainbow of colors—dark green, such as broccoli, kale, and spinach; orange, such as carrots, pumpkin, and sweet potatoes; yellow, such as yellow peppers and butternut squash.

- **Make half your grains whole.** When selecting cereals, breads, crackers, or pastas, look to see that the grains listed on the ingredient list are "whole." Whole grains provide a great source of fiber and can help in managing weight and controlling constipation.

- **Keep it lean.** Choose lean meats, fish, and poultry and bake, broil, or grill whenever possible. Try to vary your protein choices and add or substitute beans, peas, lentils, nuts, and seeds to what you eat.

- **Calcium counts.** Include 3 cups of low-fat or fat-free milk, yogurt, or equivalent of low-fat cheeses every day to maintain good bone health. Calcium-fortified foods and beverages can help fill the gap if you don't or can't consume milk.

- **Limit your fat, sugar, and salt.** These "extras" can add up! Check out the nutrition label on foods and look for foods low in saturated and trans fats. Sugars often only provide added calories with little added nutritional value. Choose and prepare foods with little salt or sodium.

Meeting the Challenges of Changing a Diet

Good nutrition is the goal, but food is not just about nutrition. It is about emotions, culture, and being social. What and how we eat is so personal that changing eating habits can be difficult. Special diets and drastic fitness programs sometimes promise the quick fix, or even the cure. Yet, the best advice for survivors is the same as for everyone: Eat a low-fat diet with a variety of grains, vegetables, and fruits, along with some high-protein foods like meat or dairy products; and balance how many calories you take in with physical activity.

Deciding to change is the first step. But the changes don't have to take place overnight. Start with the easy ones. Then, one by one, add more kinds of vegetables, reduce portion sizes, start eating more low-fat foods.

Here's a checklist for you and your survivor:

- Be realistic. Make small changes over time. Small steps can work better than giant leaps.

- Be daring and try new foods.

- Be flexible. Balance food intake with physical activity over several days. Don't focus on just one meal or one day.

- Be sensible and practice not overdoing it.

- Be active and choose activities that you enjoy and that fit into the rest of your life.

Special Needs and Considerations

Good nutrition is necessary for everyone, but sometimes things can get in the way of eating right. Ask the nurse, doctor, or pharmacist if any of the medications the person in your care is taking have possible side effects that can interfere with appetite or affect the absorption of important vitamins and minerals.

Here are some tips to ensure that the person in your care gets the nutrition he or she needs when fatigue becomes a problem.

- The thought of three big meals may be too much for the person. In fact, five to six smaller mini-meals throughout the day may be easier to manage and help keep energy levels high. Keep the fridge and pantry filled with items that provide the nutrition the person in your care needs for good health and watch those that provide little to the diet except calories. Some healthful choices can include reduced-fat cheese sticks, nuts and nut butter, fresh or dried fruit, hard-boiled eggs, low-fat yogurt or cottage cheese, bagged salads, and cut raw vegetables.

- Keep meal preparation simple. Focus on one part of the meal, like the main dish and rely on quick-cooking grains, easy-to-heat veggies and a whole-grain roll for side dishes. Save energy by collecting all the ingredients and cooking utensils first and sit down at the counter or table to put it all together.

- When you cook, try to make more than is needed for one meal. Store or freeze the rest in oven- or microwave-ready containers for quick reheating.

- Make the most of the freezer. Stock up on low-fat dinners that can be quickly reheated.

- Save menus from places that deliver healthful meals.

Changes in mobility. If eating habits remain the same while activity drops off, *weight gain* can result. Added weight can increase fatigue, further limit mobility, put a strain on the respiratory and circulatory systems (lungs, heart, blood, blood vessels), and increase the risk of other chronic illnesses. Ask a registered dietitian to recommend an ideal weight and reasonable daily calorie intake to maintain that weight. To get weight under control, pair exercise with healthy eating.

Additionally, inadequate physical activity, lack of weight-bearing exercise, and an increasingly sedentary lifestyle can result from changes in mobility that can contribute to the risk of developing *osteoporosis*—a condition where bones can become thin and fragile. While building strong bones started early in childhood, keeping them healthy as we grow older requires attention and care. Good nutrition—particularly daily sources of calcium—is important for maintaining bone health.

- Choose nonfat or low-fat dairy products often.

- Eat any type of fish with edible bones, such as canned salmon or sardines.

- Choose dark-green vegetables like kale, broccoli, turnip greens, and mustard greens. The calcium in these veggies is better absorbed than the calcium found in spinach, rhubarb, beet greens, and almonds.

- Calcium-fortified tofu, soymilk, orange juice, breads, and cereals are excellent staples. Check the food labels to see just how much calcium has been added.

- Vitamin D also plays an important role in bone health by helping with the calcium absorption. Our bodies can make vitamin D with just 15–20 minutes of skin exposure to the sun each day. Vitamin D can also be found fortified in foods that contain calcium. Be careful with supplementation because vitamin D is stored in the body and can be toxic in relatively low amounts (>2,000 i.u./day)

Eating and emotions. Depression can affect people's appetite in different ways. Many people turn to certain foods for comfort when they are depressed. These may be old favorites from childhood—a scoop of mashed potatoes, macaroni and cheese, a bowl of rice pudding. The danger is in overdoing it. These foods are often high in fat, sugar, and calories that can easily add up. On the other hand, some people lose their appetite when they are depressed. Eating with others can help you and the person in your care stay connected. Remember also that being physically active can help decrease the symptoms of depression.

Bladder problems are another issue. Quite often, fear of having to go to the bathroom frequently or loss of bladder control causes a person to limit fluids. This can cause other problems such as dehydration, dry mouth, difficulty swallowing, loss of appetite, and constipation. Find ways to fit in fluids.

- Take water breaks during the day.

- Have a beverage with meals.

- "Water down" your meals and snacks.

- Take a drink when you pass a water fountain.

- Travel with your own personal supply of bottled water.

Bowel management often involves preventing constipation. Fiber counts . . . add it up. Fiber is found in cereal, grains, nuts, seeds, vegetables, and fruit. It is not completely digested (broken down) or absorbed (taken in) by the body. A diet rich in fiber (about 25 to 30 grams each day) along with adequate fluid intake and physical activity can help promote good bowel function. Fiber can also provide a sense of fullness, which helps in managing how much one eats.

Exercise as Part of Life

Physical activity and good nutrition are perfect partners in good health. This winning combination finds a balance between what one eats and one's daily activities. Together they help in managing weight and providing energy. Physical activity not only burns calories, but it can also help the person in your care by doing the following:

- Make the most of muscle strength, or even build strength, depending on the program.

- Slowly increase the ability to do more for longer periods of time.

- Increase range of motion and joint flexibility (the ability to move easily).

- Strengthen the heart.

- Decrease feelings of fatigue.

- Decrease symptoms of depression.

- Maintain regular bowel and bladder functions.

- Cut down on the risk of skin breakdown and irritation.

- Protect weight-bearing bone mass (spine, hips, legs).

Aerobic activities raise the heart rate and breathing, and promote cardiovascular (heart and lung) fitness. Other activities develop strength and flexibility. For example, lifting weights develops strength and can help maintain good bone health. Activities like yoga and gentle stretching can improve flexibility.

Some key points to remember:

- You and the person in your care should talk with the doctor about exercise, target weight, and special needs. If possible, get a referral to a physical therapist to help begin the program.

- An exercise program needs to match the abilities and limitations of the individual. A physical therapist who has worked with survivors can design a well-balanced exercise program. With some changes, people at all levels of disability can enjoy the benefits of exercise.

- The person in your care should commit to doing what he or she can do on a consistent basis. Choosing activities you both enjoy will help you stick to your fitness plan.

- Start slowly. If the person in your care hasn't been active, begin at a low level of intensity for short periods. Alternate brief periods of exercise with periods of rest until the person in your care begins to build up endurance. Gradually increase how hard you are exercising and the length of time you are doing it.

- Join a group! Exercising with others may give you the motivation and support to keep going.

Get Moving

In addition to the diet prescription, your survivor may have gotten an exercise prescription. In general, stroke does not improve a survivor's ability to get exercise of any kind. Nonetheless, it is more important than ever that survivors participate in some form of calorie-burning activity if at all possible.

> **NOTE** A person begins to get aerobic benefit from exercise when his heart rate hits 50 percent of its maximum. No one should exceed 80 percent of his maximum heart rate during exercise.
>
> To figure maximum heart rate, subtract age from 220. For example, maximum heart rate for a 60-year-old person is 160. For aerobic benefit, he must get the heart rate up to 80 beats per minute and should not exceed 130 beats per minute.

For many stroke survivors, because of age or level of debility, the standard exercise prescription of 30 minutes most days of the week is simply not possible. So understand from the beginning, the survivor's activity level won't look like a healthy person's.

In Water

For survivors who have some weakness on one side of the body, water exercises are a good alternative because the affected side floats and feels lighter in water. Using a kickboard or simply walking in place in water may produce aerobic benefit. Water also resists movement so it produces increased heart rate in less time. Water can also be a good place to exercise for survivors with balance problems. Talk to your physical therapist about whether a water aerobics class might be appropriate for the person in your care.

> *Tip* YMCAs often offer water aerobics classes that your survivor might participate in.

On Land

Aerobic exercise on land for survivors is more problematic. The full weight of the affected side is obvious and presents balance problems and increases the danger of falling.

A readily available option for survivors with this deficit is chair exercises. These allow the survivor to remain seated while providing aerobic benefit.

> There are several DVD and video products that have complete workouts. In your search engine, type "chair exercises" or "chair dancing."

Another option for survivors with one-sided weakness or even paralysis, is an exercise machine called a seated stepper. These machines allow survivors to sit upright and move both legs and arms. (Moving arms and legs simultaneously is the most efficient way to increase heart rate and burn calories.) When seated, survivors don't have to worry about balance, as they would on a stationary bike, stair stepper, or treadmill. The survivor's feet are held in place by Velcro straps, so even if one leg is affected, the survivor can still use the machine. An affected hand can be Velcro-wrapped to one of the arm poles so that it moves back and forth. This allows survivors with moderate to severe deficits to get an aerobic workout.

> If your local health club or YMCA doesn't have a seated stepper machine, suggest they buy one. All their older members will appreciate it.

Weight Training

After stroke, muscles often weaken as a result of not being used. Weight training can be a major help in restoring these muscles. Using weights after stroke is still not common in therapy, but recent research indicates that targeted strength training in patients with muscle weakness caused by stroke significantly increased muscle power without any negative effects.

Do not take your survivor to the weight room and just leave her there. She will need supervision and instruction. Most physical trainers do not have enough special training to work with stroke survivors, but increasingly it is possible to find special needs strength trainers who may be able to help. For a basic special needs weight workout, visit www.progressiverecovery.com.

Fear of Falling

Balance is often affected by stroke, and consequently many survivors fear falling, with good reason. About 40 percent of survivors have serious falls in the first year after stroke. If your survivor has balance problems, dizziness, or a spinning sensation, see if you can get a therapy prescription from your doctor.

To reduce fear of falling, therapists often have survivors practice getting up from a lying position. This increases confidence that they can get up if they fall.

Tip To improve balance at home, bring a chair to the corner of a room. While the survivor stands in the corner, he can hold on to the back of the chair and practice moving shoulders and hips together from side to side and then forward and backward. This forces the survivor to use and strengthen the affected side.

Remember, before starting any type of workout routine, get advice from your physician. Also ask your survivor's physical therapist for suggestions. Start slowly with only moderate effort. Give the survivor time to build strength and stamina. Any amount of exercise helps reduce risk, and the benefits of exercise are cumulative, so find a way to make it easy to get exercise, that way the survivor is more likely to do it. Exercise is a particularly effective way to reduce depression.

And finally, everything said here about the benefits of aerobic exercise and weight training also applies to the caregiver. *You* need exercise as much as the person in your care. Find a way to make it part of most days.

Motivation

Motivation is the #1 factor determining whether survivors change their lifestyles or fail to follow their exercise and diet prescriptions. While motivation is an inside job, the caregiver has a part to play. Do what you can to make exercise fun. Make the new diet an experiment. If you make either diet or exercise too important, any failure becomes that much more significant. Keep it light hearted, maintain a sense of humor, and join in as much as possible.

No single day of exercise or eating right makes much of a difference in yours or your survivor's health, but 30 days does. Sixty days makes even more of an impact; a year's worth of a new lifestyle will provide remarkable shifts of biomarkers (a specific physical trait used to measure the effects or progress of a disease or condition; thinning hair is an example of a biomarker for aging), mood, and self-esteem. Survivors who take up the challenge presented by diet and exercise prescriptions make huge strides in their physical and emotional recovery; imagine what it does to their independence.

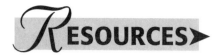

RESOURCES

American Dietetic Association
(800) 366-1655
Call weekdays 10:00 a.m. to 5:00 p.m. EST to locate a registered dietitian in your area.

Area Agency on Aging or the Cooperative Extension Service
Your local office offers free counseling by a registered dietitian.

Meals-on-Wheels
Can provide nutritious meals delivered to the home.

MyPyramid
www.mypyramid.gov
This replaces the old Food Guide Pyramid. It is a very interactive site to help people make healthy choices consistent with the 2005 Dietary Guidelines for Americans.

The National Sports Center for the Disabled (NSCD)
P.O. Box 1290
Winter Park, CO 80482
(970) 726-1540
www.nscd.org
E-mail: info@nscd.org
NSCD is a nonprofit corporation that offers winter and summer recreation. Winter sports include snow skiing, snowshoeing, and cross-country skiing. Summer recreation activities include fishing, hiking, rock climbing, whitewater rafting, camping, mountain biking, sailing, therapeutic horseback riding, and a baseball camp.

Publication

A Modification of the Rules of Golf for Golfers
with Disabilities
United States Golf Association
P.O. Box 708
Far Hills, NJ 07931-0708
(908) 234-2300.
www.usga.org/playing/rules/golfers_with_disabilities.
html
Online publication contains permissible modifications to
the rules of golf for players who are disabled.

If you don't have access to the Internet, ask your local
library to help you locate a Web site.

Emergencies

Emergencies

K̲eep a copy of the Stroke Warning Signs (p. 14) and the Cincinnati Stroke Scale (p. 17) posted on your refrigerator and near your phone. If you notice that your survivor is showing any warning signs note the time and ask her to perform the three movements explained on the Stroke Scale. If any of these movements are abnormal according to the scale, dial 911. Don't wait for the symptoms to resolve themselves or worsen, dial 911. Remember when you're dealing with stroke, time lost is brain lost.

> **NOTE** Make sure 911 is posted on your phone or ideally is on speed-dial. Keep written driving instructions near the phone for how to get to your house. If you have a speakerphone, use the speaker when talking to the dispatcher. This way, you can follow the dispatcher's instructions while attending to the emergency.

When to Call for an Ambulance

Call for an ambulance if a person—

- becomes unconscious

- has chest pain or pressure

- has trouble breathing

- has no signs of breathing (no movement or response to touch or voice)

- is bleeding severely

- is vomiting blood or is bleeding from the rectum
- has fallen and may have broken bones
- has had a seizure
- has a severe headache and slurred speech
- has pressure or severe pain in the abdomen that does not go away

OR

- if moving the person could cause further injury
- if traffic or distance would cause a life-threatening delay in getting to the hospital
- if the person is too heavy for you to lift or help

Ambulance service is expensive and may not be covered by insurance. Use it when you believe there is an emergency.

In an emergency:

Step 1: Call 911.
Step 2: Care for the victim.

Also call 911 for emergencies involving fire, explosion, poisonous gas, fallen electrical wires, or other life-threatening situations.

NOTE If the person in your care has signed a Do Not Resuscitate (DNR) order, have it available to show the paramedics. Otherwise, they are required to initiate resuscitation (reviving the person). The order must go with the patient. The Do Not Resuscitate order *must* be with the patient at all times.

In the Emergency Room

Be sure you understand the instructions for care before leaving the emergency room. Call the patient's personal doctor as soon as possible and let him or her know about the emergency room care.

Bring to the emergency room—

- insurance policy numbers
- a list of medical problems
- a list of medications currently being taken
- the personal physician's name and phone number
- the name and number of a relative or friend of the person in your care

> We strongly suggest that you take a course in CPR from your local American Red Cross, hospital, or other agency.

Choking (Adult)

Prevention

- Avoid serving excessive alcohol.
- Make sure the person in your care has a good set of dentures to chew food properly.
- Cut the food into small pieces.
- For a person who has had a stroke, use thickening powder in liquids as directed.
- Do not encourage the person to talk while eating.
- Do not make the person laugh while eating.
- Learn the Heimlich maneuver in CPR class.

Chest Pain

Any chest pain that lasts more than a few minutes is related to the heart until proven otherwise. Call 911 IMMEDIATELY. Don't wait to see if it goes away. Danger signs include—

- pain radiating from the chest down the arms, up the neck to the jaw, and into the back

- crushing, squeezing chest pain or heavy pressure in the chest

- shortness of breath, sweating, nausea and vomiting, weakness

- bluish, pale skin

- skin that is moist

- excessive perspiration

If the person is unresponsive (no movement or response to touch or voice), call 911. Be prepared to give Rescue Breathing and start CPR.

Falls and Related Injuries

Preventive measures include—

- staying in when it is rainy or icy outside

- having regular vision screening check-ups for correct eyeglasses

- using separate reading glasses and other regular glasses if bifocals make it difficult to see the floor

- being cautious when walking on wet floors

- wearing good foot support when walking

- being aware that new shoes are slippery and crepe-soled shoes can cause the toe to catch

- having foot pain problems corrected
- keeping toenails trimmed and feet healthy for good balance

A good way to tell if a part of the body has been injured in a fall is to compare it with an uninjured part. For example, compare the injured leg with the uninjured leg. Do they look and feel the same? Do they move the same way?

When you suspect a **broken bone,** follow these steps:

- If the person **cannot** move or use the injured limb, keep it from moving. Do not straighten a deformed arm or leg. Splint an injury in the position you find it.

- Support the injured part above and below the site of the injury by using folded towels, blankets, pillows, or magazines.

- If the person is face down, roll him over with the "log rolling" technique (see illustration). If you have no one to help you and the victim is breathing adequately, leave the person in the same position.

- If the person does not complain of neck pain but is feeling sick to the stomach, turn the person on one side.

- If the person complains of neck pain, keep his neck steady by putting a few pillows on either side of his head. Keep the head flat.

- Place a piece of cloth on the injury site and apply ice over the cloth.

- Keep the person warm with a blanket and make the person as comfortable as possible.

- Make a splint with cardboard or rolled-up newspaper.

▶ *Log rolling technique—
Turning a person safely
from the stomach
onto the back.*

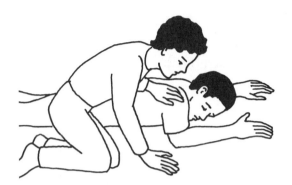
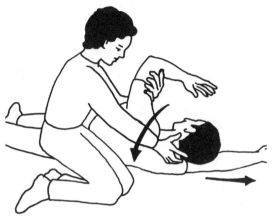

NOTE ▶ If an arm or shoulder is splinted, you might consider transporting the person by car. For neck, hip, thigh, back, and pelvic injuries, use an ambulance because the person needs to lie flat.

Checklist **Home First Aid Kit**

Buy or make a home first-aid kit. Note on the box the date when the item was purchased. Check and replenish your supplies at least once a year. These should include the following:

✓ antibiotic ointment

✓ Band-Aids®

✓ disinfectant for cleaning wounds

✓ disposable gloves

✓ emergency telephone numbers

✓ eye pads

✓ instant ice packs

✓ list of current medications

✓ pocket mask/face mask

✓ rolled gauze and elastic bandages

✓ scissors

✓ sterile gauze bandages (nonstick 4"×4")

✓ syrup of ipecac

✓ thermometer

✓ tongue depressors

✓ 3-ounce rubber bulb to rinse out wounds

✓ triangle bandage

✓ tweezers and needle

Body Mechanics—Positioning, Moving, and Transfers

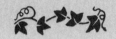

Body Mechanics—Positioning, Moving, and Transfers

Body Mechanics for the Caregiver

Body mechanics involves standing and moving one's body so as to prevent injury, avoid fatigue, and make the best use of strength. When you learn how to control and balance your own body, you can safely control and move another person. Back injuries to nursing home aides are common, so when doing any lifting be sure to use proper body mechanics.

General Rules

- Never lift more than you can comfortably handle.

- Create a base of support by standing with your feet 8–12″ (shoulder width) apart with one foot a half step ahead of the other.

Proper foot position ▶

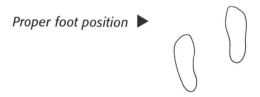

- DO NOT let your back do the heavy work—USE YOUR LEGS. (The back muscles are not your strongest muscles.)

- If the bed is low, put one foot on a footstool. This relieves pressure on your lower back.

- Consider using a support belt for your back.

Helpful Caregiver Advice for Moving a Person

These pointers are for the *caregiver* only. Be sure to see the following pages for the steps for a specific move or transfer.

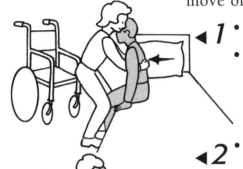

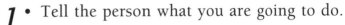

◀ 1
- Tell the person what you are going to do.
- Before starting a move, count with the person, "1-2-3."

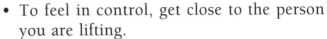

◀ 2
- To feel in control, get close to the person you are lifting.
- While lifting, keep your back in a neutral position (arched normally, not stiff), knees bent, weight balanced on both feet. Tighten your stomach and back muscles to maintain a correct support position.
- Use your arms to support the person.
- Again, *let your legs do the lifting.*

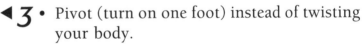

◀ 3
- Pivot (turn on one foot) instead of twisting your body.
- Breathe deeply.
- Keep your shoulders relaxed.
- When a lot of assistance is needed with transfers, tie a strong belt or a transfer belt around the person's waist and hold it as you complete the transfer.

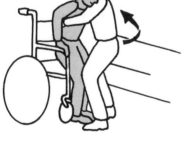

Prevention of Back and Neck Injuries

To prevent injuries to yourself, get plenty of rest and maintain:

- good nutrition
- physical fitness

- good body mechanics
- a program for managing stress

Common Treatments for Caregiver Back Pain

If you *do* experience back pain:

- Apply a cold ice pack to the injured area for 10 minutes every hour (you can use a bag of frozen vegetables).
- Get short rest periods in a comfortable position.
- Stand with your feet about shoulder width apart and hands on hips, bend backwards. Do 3–5 repetitions several times a day.
- Take short, frequent walks on a level surface.
- Avoid sitting for long periods because sitting is one of the worst healing positions.

As the caregiver, you should seek training from a physical therapist to provide this type of care so as to reduce the risk of injury to yourself or the person in your care. The therapist will correct any mistakes you make and can take into account special problems. To determine the best procedure for you to use, the therapist will consider the physical condition of the person you care for and the furniture and room arrangements in the home.

Moving a Person

When you have to move someone—either in bed or out of bed—remember these tips:

- Plan the move and know what you can and cannot do.
- Let the person do as much work as he is capable of.
- Avoid letting the person put his arms around your neck or grab you.

- Use a transfer belt to balance and support the person.

- Place transfer surfaces (wheelchair and bed) close together.

- Check wheelchair position, **brakes locked**, armrests and footrests swung out of the way.

- Let the person look to the place where he is being transferred.

- If the person is able, place his hands on the bed or chair so he can assist in the movement. If the person has had a stroke or is afraid, have him clasp his hands close to his chest.

- Ask the person to *push* rather than *pull* on the bed rails, the chair, or you.

- Work at the person's level and speed and check for pain.

- Avoid sudden jerking motions.

- Never pull on the person's arms or shoulders.

- Correctly position the person. (This helps the body regain lost function and helps prevent additional function loss.)

- Have the person wear shoes with good treads or sturdy slippers.

 To encourage independence, let the person assist as he is able. It's okay for the person to stand up partly and sit back down.

Positioning a Person in Bed

1 ▶

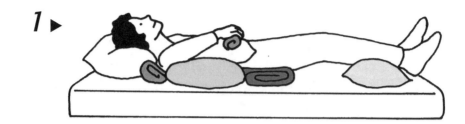

- Place a small pillow under the person's head, keeping his spine neutral.

- Place a small pillow lengthwise under the calf of the weak leg, let the heel hang off the end of the pillow to prevent pressure, and loosen the top sheet to avoid pressure on the toes.

2 ▶

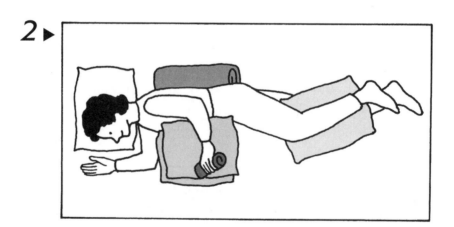

- Fold a bath towel under the hip of the person's weak side.

- Place the weak arm and elbow on a pillow higher than the heart.

Positioning a Person on His or Her Strong Side

1. Place a small pillow under the person's head.

2. Keep the person's head in alignment with the spine.

3. Place a rolled pillow at the back to prevent rolling.

4. Place a pillow in front to keep the arm the same height as the shoulder joint.

5. Place a medium pillow lengthwise between the knees, legs, and ankles. (The person's knees may be bent slightly.)

Positioning a Person on His or Her Weak Side

1. Use the same positioning as described above.

2. Change the person's position frequently because he may not be aware of pressure, pain, or skin irritation.

Moving a person in bed can injure the person in care or the caregiver if certain basic rules are not followed:

- Never grab or pull the person's arm or leg.

- If the medical condition allows, raise the foot of the bed slightly to prevent the person from sliding down.

- If moving him is difficult, get him out of bed and back in the wheelchair and start over by putting him in bed closer to the headboard.

Moving a Person Up in Bed

1. Tell the person what you are going to do.

2. Lower the head of the bed to a flat position and remove the pillow—never try to move the person "uphill."

3. If possible, raise the bed and **lock the wheels**.

4. Tell the person to bend his knees and brace his feet firmly against the mattress to help push.

5. Stand at the side of the bed and place one hand behind the person's back and the other underneath the buttocks.

6. Bend your knees and keep your back in a neutral position.

7. Count "1-2-3" and have the person push with his feet and pull with his hands toward the head of the bed.

8. Replace the pillow under his head.

Using Two People to Move an Unconscious Person

1
- Tell the person what you are going to do even if the person seems to be unconscious.

- Remove the pillow.

- If possible, raise the bed and **lock the wheels**.

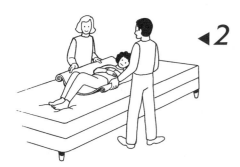

◀*2*
- Stand on either side of the bed.

- Face the head of the bed, with feet 8–12″ apart, knees bent, back in a neutral position.

- Roll the sides of the draw sheet up to the person's body.

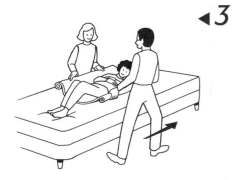

◀*3*
- Grab the draw sheet with your palms up.

- Count "1-2-3" and then shift your body weight from the back to the front leg, keeping your arms and back in a locked position. Together, slide the person smoothly up the bed.

- Replace pillows under the person's head.

- Position the person comfortably.

A draw sheet—a sheet folded several times and positioned under the person to be moved in bed—prevents irritation to his skin. The sheet should be positioned from the shoulders to just below the knees.

Moving an Unconscious Person Alone

1. If possible, raise the whole bed and **lock the wheels**.

2. Remove the pillow.

3. Face the front of the bed, with feet 8–12″ apart, knees bent, back in a neutral position.

4. Roll the edge of the draw sheet and grab it.

5. Slide your arms under the draw sheet and the person's shoulders and back.

6. Count "1-2-3" and then shift your body weight from your back to front leg, keeping your arms and back in a locked position.

7. Slide the person to the top of the bed.

8. Replace the pillow.

9. Position the person comfortably.

 PREVENTING BACK INJURIES
Having the person grab a trapeze to help with the move is easiest and safest for your back. (📖 See p. 135.)

Moving the Person to One Side of the Bed on His or Her Back

1 • Place your feet 8–12″ apart, knees bent, back in a neutral position.

   • Slide your arms under the person's back to her far shoulder blade. (Bend your knees and hips to lower yourself to the person's level.)

   • Slide the person's shoulders toward you by rocking your weight to your back foot.

2 • Use the same procedure at the person's buttocks and feet.

   • Always keep your knees bent and your back in a neutral position.

1 ▼

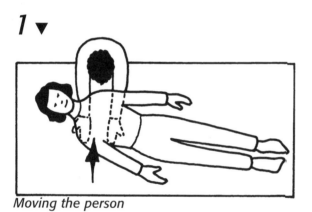

Moving the person

2 ▼

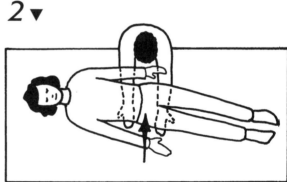

Rolling Technique

1. Move the person to one side of the bed as in the above procedure.

2. Bend the person's knees.

3. Hold the person at her hip and shoulder blade on the far side of the body.

4. Roll the person *toward* you to make sure she does not fall off the bed.

Raising the Person's Head and Shoulders

1. If possible, ask the person to lift her head and dig both elbows into the bed to support her body.

2. Face the head of the bed, feet 8–12″ apart, knees bent, back in neutral.

3. Help the person lift her shoulders by placing your hands and forearms under the pillow and her shoulder blades.

4. Use bent knees, back in neutral, and locked arms to assist the lift.

5. Adjust the pillow.

Helping a Person Sit Up

1. Tell the person what you are going to do.

2. Bend the person's knees.

3. Roll her on her side so she is facing you.

4. Reach one arm under her shoulder blade.

5. Place the other arm in back of her knees.

6. Position your feet 8–12″ apart with your center of gravity close to the bed and the person.

7. Keep your back in a neutral position.

8. Count "1-2-3" and shift your weight to your back leg.

9. Shift the person's legs over the edge of the bed while pulling her shoulders to a sitting position.

10. Remain in front of her until she is stabilized.

Transfers

Transferring a person in and out of bed is an important caregiver activity. It can be done fairly easily if these instructions are followed. Use the same procedure for all transfers so that a routine is set up.

Transfers Using a Mechanical Lift

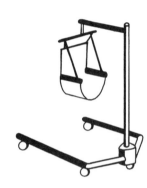

1. Tell the person what you are going to do.
2. Place the chair next to the bed with the back of the chair in line with the headboard of the bed. **Lock the wheels**.
3. Place a blanket or sheet over the chair.
4. Turn the person on one side toward the edge of the bed.
5. Fan-fold a sling and place it at the person's back.
6. Roll her to her other side, pull the sling out flat, and center it under her body.
7. Attach the sling to the mechanical lift with the hooks in place and facing out through the metal frame.
8. Fold the person's arms across her chest.
9. Using the crank, lift her out of bed.
10. Guide the legs. Lower her onto the chair.
11. Remove the hooks from the frame of the mechanical lift.
12. Leave the person in the chair with the sling under her, comfortably adjusted.
13. To get the person back in the bed, put the hooks facing out through the metal frame of the sling.
14. Raise the person using the crank.
15. Guide her legs. Lower her onto the bed.

16. Remove the hooks from the frame.

17. Remove the sling from under the person by turning her from side to side on the bed.

18. Properly position her with pillows. (📖 See p. 294.)

For lift instructions and precautions, refer to the *Positioning and Transfer Guide* that comes with your mechanical lift.

Helping a Person Stand

Help only as much as needed but guard the person from falling.

1. Have her sit on the edge of the chair or bed. Let her rest a moment if she feels lightheaded.

2. Instruct her to push off with her hands from the bed or chair armrests.

3. Position your knee between her knees.

4. Face her and support the weak knee against one or both of your knees as needed.

5. Put your arms around the person's waist or use a transfer belt.

6. Keep your back in a neutral position.

7. At the count of "1-2-3," instruct the person to stand up while pulling her toward you and pushing your knees into her knee if needed.

8. Once she is upright, have her keep her knee locked straight.

9. Support and balance her as needed.

NOTE ▷ If during a transfer you start to "lose" the person, do not try to hold her up. Instead, lower her to the floor.

Helping a Person Sit

1. Reverse the process described in Helping a Person Stand.

2. Direct the person to feel for the chair or bed with the back of the legs.

3. Direct the person to reach back with both hands to the bed or chair armrests and slowly sit.

Transferring from Bed to Wheelchair with a Transfer Belt

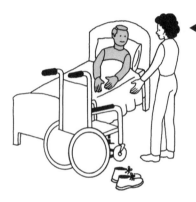

◄ **1** • Place the wheelchair at a 45° angle to the bed so that the person will be transferring to his stronger side.

• **Lock the wheels** of the chair and the bed.

• Tell the person what you are going to do.

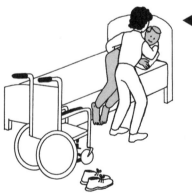

◄ **2** • Put on his shoes while he is still lying down if he is weak or unstable.

• Bring him to a sitting position with his legs over the edge of the bed.

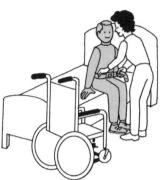

◀ **3** • Let him rest a moment if he feels lightheaded.

• Use a **transfer belt** for a person needing a lot of support.

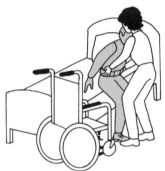

◀ **4** • Bring him to a standing position as described on page 301.

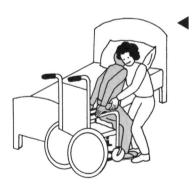

◀ **5** • Have him reach for the chair arm and pivot. A very fast pivot may frighten the person, or cause you to lose knee control and fall with a person who is totally dependent.

• Support him with your arms and knees as needed.

• Adjust him comfortably in the chair.

NOTE ▷ If the person starts to slide off the edge of the bed before or after the transfer, lay his upper torso across the bed to prevent him from falling to the floor.

Transferring from Wheelchair to Bed

1. Reverse the process described in Transfer from Bed to Wheelchair.

2. Place the chair at a 45° angle to the bed so the person is on his stronger side. **Lock the wheels**.

3. Get into a position to provide a good base of support; use good body mechanics.

4. Have the person stand, reach for the bed, and pivot.

5. Support and guide him as needed.

6. Adjust the person in bed with pillows.

Transferring from Bed to Wheelchair Without a Transfer Belt

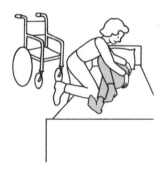

- Place the wheelchair at a 45° angle to the bed so that the person will be transferring to his stronger side.

- **Lock the wheels** of the chair (you can use a wheel block) and the wheels of the bed.

- Tell the person what you are going to do.

- Bring him to a sitting position with his legs over the edge of the bed following steps a, b, c, and d.

1a ▲

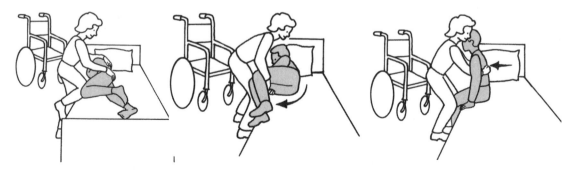

1b ▲   *1c* ▲   *1d* ▲

- Let him rest a moment if he feels lightheaded.
- Put his shoes on.

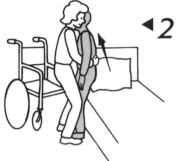

◀ **2** • Put your arms around his chest and clasp your hands behind his back.
- Support the leg that is farther from the wheelchair between your legs.

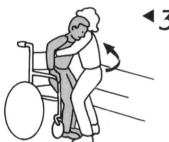

◀ **3** • Lean back, shift your leg, and lift.
- Pivot toward the chair.

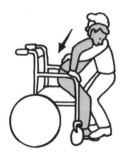

◀ **4** • Bend your knees and let him bend toward you.
- Lower the person into the wheelchair.
- Adjust him comfortably in the chair.

NOTE As the person becomes stronger, you can provide less assistance. However, use the same body positioning to support the person's weaker side.

Transferring from Wheelchair to Bed with a Transfer Board

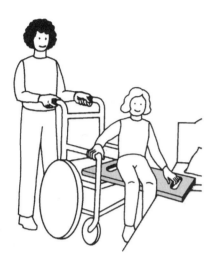

1. As much as possible, make the bed and the chair the same height.

2. Place the wheelchair at a 45° angle to the bed so that the person will be transferring to her stronger side.

3. **Lock the wheels** of the chair (you can use a wheel block) and the wheels of the bed.

4. Tell the person what you are going to do.

5. Remove the armrest nearest the bed.

6. Remove her feet from the footrests and swing the footrests out of the way.

7. Have the person lift her hip and place the board under the hip with the other end of the board on the bed.

8. MAKE SURE SHE DOESN'T PUT HER FINGERS UNDER THE BOARD.

9. Ask her to put her hands on the board with the hands close to her sides.

10. Ask her to lean slightly forward and to make a series of small pushes off the board by straightening her elbows and inching along the board toward the bed.

11. When she is on the bed, ask her to lean over onto her elbow and pull the transfer board out from under her bottom.

12. Adjust her comfortably in the bed.

Transferring from a Wheelchair to a Car

Be sure the car is parked on a level surface without cracks or potholes.

1 • Open the passenger door as far as possible.

• Move the left side of the wheelchair as close to the car seat as possible.

• **Lock the chair's wheels**.

• Move both footrests out of the way.

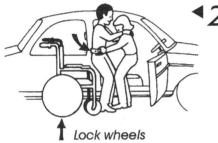

↑ *Lock wheels*

◀*2* • Position yourself facing the person.

• Tell him what you are going to do.

• Bending your knees and hips, lower yourself to his level.

• By grasping the transfer belt around his waist help him stand while straightening your hips and knees.

• If his legs are weak, brace his knees with your knees.

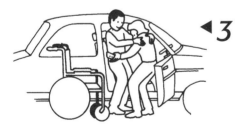

◀*3* • While he is standing, turn him so he can be eased down to sit on the car seat. GUIDE HIS HEAD so it is not bumped.

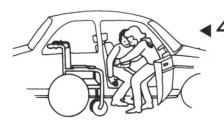

◀*4* • Lift his legs into the car by putting your hands under his knees.

• Move him to face the front.

• Put on his seat belt.

• Close door carefully.

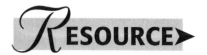

American Academy of Orthopaedic Surgeons
6300 N. River Road
Rosemont, IL 60018
(800) 346-AAOS (800-346-2267)
www.aaos.org
Offers a free booklet Lift It Safe *on lifting procedures for home-based carergivers.*

If you don't have access to the Internet, ask your local library to help you locate a Web site.

Part Three: Additional Resources

Chapter

Common Abbreviations

Acute MI – heart attack

ADA – Americans with Disabilities Act

ADL – activities of daily living

AFO – ankle-foot orthosis

ALF – assisted living facility

ASHD – arteriosclerotic heart disease

BC – blood culture

BID – 2 times per day (approximately 8 and 8 as medication times)

BP – blood pressure

BRP – bathroom privileges

BS – blood sugar

C&S – culture and sensitivity

CA – cancer/carcinoma

CABG – coronary artery bypass graft

CBC – complete blood count

CCU – coronary care unit

CHF – congestive heart failure

CNS – central nervous system

COPD – chronic obstructive pulmonary disease

CPR – cardiopulmonary resuscitation

CSF – cerebrospinal fluid

CVA – cerebral vascular accident

CVD – cerebral vascular disease

DM – diabetes mellitus

DME – durable medical equipment

DRG – diagnosis related group

Dx – diagnosis

ED – emergency department

EDSS – Expanded Disability Status Scale

EEG – electroencephalogram recording of the brain's electrical activity

EKG/ECG – electrocardiogram recording of the heart's electrical activity

EP – evoked potential

FBS – fasting blood sugar, or the amount of glucose in the blood when a person has not eaten for 12 hours

FX – fracture

GTT – glucose tolerance test to determine a person's ability to metabolize glucose

HC – home care

HHA – a home health agency providing home health services

HS – hour of sleep (medication time)

I&O – record of food and liquid taken in and waste eliminated

ICU – intensive care unit for special monitoring of the acutely ill

IV – intravenous line to drip fluids and blood products into the bloodstream

LOC – loss of consciousness

MCD – Medicaid

MCR – Medicare

MRI – magnetic resonance imaging

MS – multiple sclerosis

Neuro – neurologist

NPO – nothing by mouth

NSAID – nonsteroid anti-inflammatory drug.

OBS – organic brain syndrome, an injury or disorder that interferes with normal brain function

OR – operating room

OT – occupational therapy or occupational therapist

PO – by mouth

Psych – psychiatric; psychologist

PT – physical therapy or physical therapist

QID – 4 times per day (approximately 9–1–5–9 as medication times)

RBC – red blood count

RN – nurse

ROM – range of motion

RR – respiratory rate

RT – recreational therapy

Rx – prescription

SLP – speech–language pathologist

SNF – skilled nursing facility

SOB – shortness of breath

SS or SSA – Social Security or Social Security Administration

SSI/SSDI – supplemental security income or diability income

ST – Speech therapist or speech therapy

Sx – symptoms

TIA – transient ischemic attack

TID – 3 times per day (approximately 9–1–6 as medication times)

TPN – total parenteral nutrition

TPR – temperature, pulse, respiration

TX – treatment

U/A – urine analysis

VEP – visual evoked potential

VNS – visiting nurse service

WBC – white blood count

Common Specialists

Allergist/Immunologist
Disorders of the immune system

Anesthesiologist
Pain relief during and after surgery

Audiologist
Hearing disorders

Cardiologist
Conditions of the heart, lungs, and blood vessels

Chiropodist
Minor foot ailments such as corns and bunions

Colon and Rectal Surgeon
Diseases of the intestinal tract

Dentist
Teeth and gums

Dermatologist
Skin, hair, and nails

Endocrinologist
Hormonal problems including thyroid disorders

Forensic psychiatrist
Behavior assessment for legal purposes

Gastroenterologist
Digestive system, stomach, liver, bowels, and gallbladder

Geriatric psychiatrist
Emotional disorders of elderly persons

Geriatrician
Disorders common to elderly persons

Gynecologist
Female reproductive system

Hematologist
Diseases of the blood, spleen, and lymph glands

Internist
Primary care of common illnesses, both long term and emergency

Nephrologist
Kidney diseases and disorders

Neurologist
Brain and nervous system disorders

Nurse Practitioner
Provides preventive and medical health care in association with a physician

Oncologist
All cancers

Ophthalmologist
Care and surgery of the eyes

Optician
Fitting and making of eyeglasses and contact lenses

Optometrist
Basic eye care

Oral maxillofacial surgeon
Surgery involving the teeth, gums, and jaw

Orthopedist
Surgery involving joints, bones, and muscles

Orthotist
Nonmedical specialist in the measurement, sizing, and preparation of foot padding pieces

Osteopath (DO)
General medicine with emphasis on the promotion of health through the hands-on manipulation of the muscles, tendons, and joints

Otolaryngologist
Head and neck surgeon

Pharmacist
Medications specialist; provider of physician and patient education

Physiatrist
Rehabilitation asessment and planning

Podiatrist
Foot care

Psychiatrist (MD)
Emotional, mental, or addictive disorders

Psychologist (MA or PhD)
Assessment and care of emotional or mental disorders

Pulmonologist
Diseases of lungs and airways

Rheumatologist
Diseases of joints and connective tissue (arthritis)

Urologist
Urinary system and the male reproductive system

Glossary

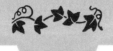

𝕾 A

Activities of daily living (ADL): personal hygiene, bathing, dressing, grooming, toileting, feeding, and transferring

Acute: state of illness that comes on suddenly and may be of short duration

Acute rehab: rehab that occurs in the first few weeks after the acute event, either in a hospital or rehab facility

Adult day care: centers that have a supervised environment where seniors can be with others

Advance directive: a legal document that states a person's health care preferences in writing while that person is competent and able to make such decisions

Ambulatory: able to walk with little or no assistance

Amnesia: complete or partial loss of memory

Analgesics: medications used to relieve pain

Antibiotics: a group of drugs used to combat infection

Anus: the opening of the rectum

Anxiety: a state of discomfort, dread, and foreboding with physical symptoms such as rapid breathing and heart rate, tension, jitteriness, and muscle aches

Aorta: the main artery leading from the heart

Apathy: a condition in which the person shows little or no emotion

Aphasia: a language disorder that affects a survivor's ability to use language; it may affect speaking, reading, writing, or comprehension

Apraxia: difficulty making purposeful movement. Verbal apraxia refers to a problem coordinating muscles necessary for speech and is different than aphasia, which is a problem with language.

Aromatherapy: use of essential oils of various plants to treat symptoms of diseases, improve sleep, and reduce stress by inducing relaxation

Artificial life-support systems: the use of respirators, tube feeding, intravenous (IV) feeding, and other means to replace natural and vital functions, such as breathing, eating, and drinking

Assessment: the process of analyzing a person's condition

Assisted living: housing for seniors offering independence, choice of services, and assistance with activities of daily living (ADLs), including meals and housekeeping

Assistive devices: any tools that are designed, fabricated, and/or adapted to assist a person in performing a particular task, e.g., cane, walker, shower chair

Assistive technology: a term used to describe all of the tools, products and devices, from the simplest to the most complex, that can make a particular function easier to perform

Atherosclerosis: a progressive disease where the blood vessels slowly become clogged with cholesterol and cellular waste. It is present in everyone but varies in intensity and is often the cause of blockage strokes.

At-home rehabilitation: rehab performed by a therapist who comes to the survivor's home

Atrial fibrillation: a disease of the heart where its upper chamber vibrates rather than contracts fully, allowing clots to form in the stalled blood. These clots can move out of the heart and into the brain. Often called "A-fib."

Atrophy: the wasting away of muscles or brain tissue

B

Bedpan: a container into which a person urinates and defecates while in bed

Blood pressure: the pressure of the blood on the walls of the blood vessels and arteries

Body language: gestures that serve as a form of communication

Body mechanics: proper use and positioning of the body to do work and avoid strain and injury

C

Calorie: the measure of the energy the body gets from various foods

Cardiovascular system: the heart and blood vessels

Carotid artery: the main artery delivering blood to the brain

Cataract: a condition (often found in the elderly) in which the lens of the eye become opaque

Catheter: a tube inserted into the bladder to collect or drain urine

Cerebellum: the part of the brain that regulates and coordinates complex voluntary muscular movement as well as the maintenance of posture and balance

Chronic: refers to a state or condition that lasts 6 months or longer

Cincinnati Stroke Scale: see FAST

Cognition: high-level functions carried out by the human brain, including comprehension and use of speech, visual perception and construction, calculation ability, attention (information processing), memory, and executive functions such as planning, problem-solving, and self-monitoring

Cognitive rehabilitation: rehabilitation, usually delivered by a speech therapist, that deals with cognitive functions like memory, judgment, impulsivity and thought sequencing

Colostomy: a temporary or permanent surgical procedure that creates an artificial opening through the abdominal wall into a part of the large bowel through which feces can leave the body

Congregate living: a type of independent living in which elderly people can live in their own apartments but have meals, laundry, transportation, and housekeeping services available

Conservator: a person given the power to take over and protect the interests of one who is incompetent

Constipation: infrequent or uncomfortable bowel movements

Contracture: shortening or tightening of the tissue around a joint so that the person loses the ability to move easily

✑ D

Decubitus ulcer: pressure sore; bedsore

Defecate: to have a bowel movement

Defibrillator: a device that uses and electrical current to restore or regulate a stopped or disorganized heartbeat

Deficit: everyday abilities that have been taken away by a stroke

Dehydration: loss of normal body fluid, sometimes caused by vomiting and severe diarrhea

Delusions: beliefs that are firmly held despite proof that they are false

Dementia: a progressive decline in mental functions

Depression: a psychiatric condition that can be moderate or severe and cause feelings of sadness and emptiness

Diuretics: drugs that help the body get rid of fluids

Draw sheet: a sheet folded widthwise to position under someone in bed to keep the linen clean and aid in transfers

Durable Power of Attorney: a legal document that authorizes another to act as one's agent and is "durable" because it remains in effect in case the person becomes disabled or mentally incompetent

Durable Power of Attorney for Health Care Decisions: a legal document that lets a person name someone else to make health care decisions after the person has become disabled or mentally incompetent and is unable to make those decisions

Dysphagia: difficulty with or abnormal swallowing

E

Edema: an abnormal swelling in legs, ankles, hands, or abdomen that occurs because the body is retaining fluids

Estate planning: a process of planning for the present and future use of a person's assets

Evoked potentials (EPs): EPs are recordings of the nervous system's electrical response to the stimulation of specific sensory pathways (e.g., visual, auditory, general sensory)

F

FAST: a stroke-diagnosis tool that is based on an acronym for facial droop, arm weakness, speech problems, and time last seen normal.

Foot drop: a condition of weakness in the muscles of the foot and ankle, caused by poor nerve conduction, which interferes with a person's ability to flex the ankle and walk with a normal heel–toe pattern; the toes touch the ground before the heel, causing the person to trip or lose balance

Foster care: a care arrangement in which a person lives in a private home with a primary caregiver and 4 or 5 other people

G

Gait: the manner in which a person walks

Geriatric: refers to care of older adults

Guardian: the one who is legally designated to have protective care of another person or of that person's property

H

Hallucination: false perceptions (usually visual) of things that are not really there

HDL: "good or healthy" cholesterol (high-density lipoprotein)

Heimlich maneuver: a method for clearing the airway of a choking person

Hemiparesis: slight paralysis or weakness affecting one side of the body

Hemiplegia: paralysis affecting only one side of the body

Hospice: a program that allows a dying person to remain at home while receiving professionally supervised care

Hypertension: blood pressure higher than 120/80

I

Incontinence: involuntary discharge of urine or feces

Interventional radiologist: a specialist who uses hi-tech imaging devices to deliver specialized treatment such as balloons, drugs, and stents for treatment of acute stroke

Intracerebral hemorrhage: a type of bleeding stroke where a blood vessel deep in the brain ruptures and blood pressing into the brain tissue destroys it

Intravenous (IV): the delivery of fluids, medications, or nutrients into a vein

L

Laxative: a substance taken by mouth to produce a bowel movement in 6–9 hours

LDL: "bad" cholesterol (low-density lipoprotein)

M

Mechanical lift: a machine used to lift a person from one place to another

Medic-Alert®: bracelet identification system linked to a 24-hour service that provides full information in the case of an emergency

Medicaid: a U.S. health program that uses state and federal funds to pay certain medical and hospital expenses of those having low income, with benefits that vary from state to state

Medicare: the federal health insurance program in the U.S. for people 65 or older and for certain people under 65 who are disabled

N

Neurologist: a doctor specializing in diagnosing and treating diseases of the brain and nervous system

Neuroradiologist: a specialist who uses radioactive substances and X-rays to diagnose disease

Neurosurgeon: a doctor specializing in brain surgery

Nutrition: a process of giving the body the key nutrients it needs for proper body function

O

Occupational therapy: therapy that focuses on the activities of daily living such as personal hygiene, bathing, dressing, grooming, toileting, and feeding

Ombudsman: a person who helps residents of a retirement or health care facility with such problems as quality of care, food, finances, medical care, residents rights, and other concerns; these services are confidential and free

Oral hygiene: the process of keeping the mouth clean

P

Paralysis: loss or impairment of voluntary movement of a group of muscles

Paranoia: a mental disorder characterized by delusions (often the belief that one is being persecuted)

Paraplegic: one who is paralyzed in (usually) the lower half of the body

Passive suicide: killing oneself through indirect action or inaction, such as no longer taking life-prolonging medications

Pathogen: a disease-causing microorganism

Perseveration: a cognitive problem where survivors can't control certain behaviors

Physiatrist: a doctor who specializes in rehabilitation

Physical therapist: a therapist who works with restoring gross motor coordination

Physical therapy: therapy that focuses on gait, transfers, massage, and adaptive equipment

Plateau: a period of time during therapy when there is little or no improvement

Posey: a vest-like restraint used to keep a person from getting out of bed

Positioning: placing a person in a position that allows functional activity and minimizes the danger of faulty posture that could cause pressure sores, impaired breathing, and shrinking of muscles and tendons

Power of Attorney for Health Care: providing another person with the authority to make health care decisions

Pressure sore: a breakdown of the skin caused by prolonged pressure in one spot; a bed sore; decubitus ulcer

Prognosis: a forecast of what is likely to happen when an individual contracts a particular disease or condition

Prone: lying facedown

Propulsion: propelling forward as the patient accelerates with rapid, short steps

Prosthesis: an artificial body part, such as a tooth, an eye, a breast, leg, arm, hand, or foot

❧ Q

Quadriplegia: paralysis of both the upper and lower parts of the body from the neck down

❧ R

Range of motion (ROM): the extent of possible passive (movement by another person) movement in a joint

Rehabilitation: after a disabling injury or disease, restoration of a person's maximum physical, mental, vocational, social, and spiritual potential

Rehabilitation psychologist: a psychologist who helps design therapy plans and who helps rehab patients deal with the emotions connected with their condition

Respite care: short-term care that allows a primary caregiver time off from his or her responsibilities

Rigidity: a tightness or increase in muscle tone at rest or throughout the entire range of motion of a limb, which may be felt as a stiffness by the patient

S

Sedatives: medications used to calm a person

Shock: a state of collapse resulting from reduced blood volume and/or blood pressure caused by burns, severe injury, pain, or an emotional blow

Sitz bath: a bath in which only the hips and buttocks are immersed into water or a medicated solution

Speech therapist: a therapist who works in the areas of speech production, language comprehension, swallowing and cognitive deficits

Speech therapy: therapy that focuses on the treatment of disorders of speech, swallowing, and communication

Stroke: sudden loss of function of a part of the brain due to interference in its blood supply, usually by hemorrhage or blood clotting

Sub-acute rehabilitation: outpatient rehab done at a facility

Subarachnoid hemorrhage: a type of bleeding stroke in which a blood vessel breaks and bleeds into the space between the brain and the skull, not into the brain itself

Supine: lying on one's back

Support groups: groups of people who get together to share common experiences and help one another cope

Symptom: sign of a disease or disorder that helps in diagnosis

T

tPA (tissue plasminogen activatior): a drug used to break up clots; the first (and currently only) FDA-approved treatment of acute stroke

Tracheotomy: surgical procedure to make an opening in a person's windpipe to aid in breathing

Tranquilizers: a class of drugs used to calm a person and control certain emotional disturbances

Transfer: movements from one position to another, for example, from bed to chair, wheelchair to car, etc.

Transfer belt: a device placed around the waist of a disabled person and used to secure the person while walking; gait belt

Transfer board (Sliding Board): polished wooden or plastic board used to slide a person when moving from one place to another, for example, bed to wheelchair or commode

Trapeze: a metal bar suspended over a bed to help a person raise up or move

U

Urinal: a container used by a bedridden male for urinating

Urinalysis: a laboratory test of urine

V

Vaginal douche: a procedure to cleanse or medicate a woman's vagina by sending a stream of water into the vaginal opening

Vital signs: life signs such as blood pressure, breathing, and pulse

Void: to urinate; pass water

W

Will: a legal document that states how to dispose of a person's property after death according to that person's wishes

Caregiver Organizations

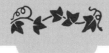

Stroke Organizations

The American Stroke Association
7272 Greenville Avenue
Dallas, TX 75231
www.StrokeAssociation.org
Stroke Family "Warmline"
(888) 4-STROKE (478-7653)

Heart and Stroke Foundation of Canada
http://ww2.heartandstroke.ca
222 Queen Street, Suite 1402
Ottawa, ON K1P 5V9
(613) 569-4361 Fax (613) 569-3278

The Stroke Association — England
http://www.stroke.org.uk/
Stroke helpline 0845 3033 100
(open Monday to Friday, 9 am to 5 pm)
E-mail: info@stroke.org.uk or write to
Stroke Information Service
The Stroke Association
240 City Road
London EC1V 2PR

The National Stroke Foundation — Australia
http://www.strokefoundation.com.au/
Level 8, 99 Queen Street
Melbourne VIC 3000
Phone 03 9670 1000 Fax 03 9670 9300
Information line - 1800 787 653 ABN 420 061 733 79

European Stroke Initiative
http://www.eusi.org/

International Caregiver Information and Support Organizations

AUSTRALIA

Carers Australia
www.carersaustralia.com.au
(800) 242-636
Carers Australia represents the needs and interests of caregivers at the national level.

CANADA

Canadian Caregiver Coalition
www.ccc-ccan.ca
The Canadian Caregivers Coalition helps identify and respond to the needs of caregivers in Canada. Links to organizations helpful to caregivers.

Caregiver Network, Inc.
(416) 323-1090
www.caregiver.on.ca
Based in Toronto, Canada, CNI's goal is to be a national single-information source to make your life as a caregiver easier.

UNITED KINGDOM

Carers UK

www.carersuk.org

The leading campaigning, policy, and information organization for carers; membership organization, led and set up by carers in 1965 to have a voice and to win the recognition and support that carers deserve.

*See **Resources** p. 183 for more caregiver support information.*

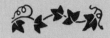

Shampooing hair, 200–203
    dry shampoo, 202
    wet shampoo, 201–202
    wet shampoo in bed, 202–203
Sharing in medical decisions, 63–65
Shaving, 189, 203–204
Shower, 199
    grab bars for, 137
Shower hose, hand-held, 137
Sight aids, 140
Skilled care facilities, 46
Skilled nursing facility, 49
Skin care, 194
    pressure sores, 226
        prevention, 222–226
        treatment, 225–226
    turning someone in bed, 225
Social Services Block Grant, 97
Speech, loss of, 244–245
Speech therapist, 61
Speech therapy, 238–239
State personal assistance program, 80
Suction catheters, 146
Summoning help, devices for, 142–143
Support groups, location of, 174
Support system, 39
Supportive housing, 44–53

Table, over-the-bed, 135
Tax rules for hiring of personal assistants, 85
Team
    for health care, 56–76 (*See also* Health care
        team)
Telephone, 124–125
Tests, questions regarding, 65–69
Therapies, 233–241
    acupuncture, 239
    occupational therapy, 238
    pet therapy, 239–240
    physical therapy, 234–237
    range-of-motion exercises, 235–237
    speech therapy, 238–239
TIAs. *See* Mini-strokes
Timing of response to stroke, 14–16
Tissue plasminogen activator, 15–16
Toilet frame, 137

Toilet seat, raised, 137
Toileting, 211–219. *See also* Activities of Daily
        Living
tPA medication. *See* Tissue plasminogen
        activator
Transfer bench, bath, 137
Transfer board, 135
Transfers, 300–307
    from bed to wheelchair
        with transfer belt, 302–303
        without transfer belt, 304–305
    helping person sit, 302
    helping person stand, 301
    mechanical lifts, 300–301
    from wheelchair to bed, 304
        with transfer board, 306
    from wheelchair to car, 307
Transient ischemic attacks, 30
Transportation services, 104
Transtracheal oxygen therapy equipment, 146
Trapeze bar, 134
Tub, grab bars for, 137
Tub bath, 198
Turning someone in bed, 225
Types of health care professionals, 84–85

Undressing, 191–193, 207
Urinal use, 135, 213
Urinary tract infection, 217

Vehicle adaptation, 250–251
Vision care, 70–71
Visit to doctor's office, 65
    preparing for, 64–65

Warning signs of stroke, 8, 14, 28
Water exercises, 274
Weakness, sudden onset of, 14
Weight loss, 263
Weight training, 275–276
Wet shampoo, 201–202
    in bed, 202–203
Wheelchairs
    attachments for, 139
    requirements, 139
Work, returning to, after stroke, 251–257